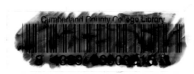

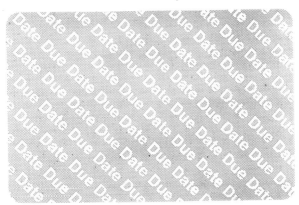

DEMCO

# The Body in Medical Culture

# The Body

## *in*

## Medical Culture

*Edited by*

Elizabeth Klaver

**SUNY**
PRESS

Published by
State University of New York Press, Albany

For information, contact State University of New York Press, Albany, NY
www.sunypress.edu

Production by Marilyn P. Semerad
Marketing by Fran Keneston

Library of Congress Cataloging-in-Publication Data

The body in medical culture / edited by Elizabeth Klaver.
    p. ; cm.
    Includes bibliographical references and index.
    ISBN 978-1-4384-2585-6 (hardcover : alk. paper) —
    ISBN 978-1-4384-2586-3 (pbk. : alk. paper)
    1. Social medicine. 2. Body, Human–Social aspects. 3. Culture. 4. Medicine—
History. I. Klaver, Elizabeth. [DNLM: 1. History of Medicine. 2. Human Body.
3. Attitude to Health. 4. Body Image. WZ 40 B668 2009]
    RA418.B5795 2009
    362.1–dc22

                                                                        2008024284

10  9  8  7  6  5  4  3  2  1

# Contents

# Illustrations

# Acknowledgments

On behalf of the authors, I would like to thank the editorial staff at SUNY Press for their assistance at every stage in the making of this book. The readers of the manuscript made particularly good suggestions, many of which were incorporated into the chapters, and I thank them for their generosity. To friends, colleagues, and students, who suggested resources and ideas to consider, you have our utmost appreciation. And to Jean Bossom and Midge Swedberg, who gave editorial assistance at a crucial moment, my gratitude. We thank the Bodleian Library, University of Oxford, Birmingham Central Library, The Harvard Theatre Collection, Houghton Library, Grand Central Publishing, and Gary J. Alter, MD, for graciously granting permission to use illustrations from their collections for chapters 3, 6, and 8.

# Introduction

## ELIZABETH KLAVER

> To enter the historical arena is to enter a world where
> we see what we assume has always been present actually
> being manufactured, being created in political circum-
> stances, in educational contexts, even in the market-
> place, where we may think doctors, in the modern sense,
> are out of place.
> —Michael Neve, *The Western Medical Tradition*

IN THE EPIGRAPH ABOVE, MICHAEL Neve is surely pointing not only to our modern assumptions about medicine, where doctors may be seen as definitely "in place," but also to a culture of medicine that is much larger and more encompassing than simply what we recognize today as the obvious venues where medicine takes place—the hospital, the clinic, the medical school, the research laboratory.[1] In fact, to think about a medical culture in the West, as this book proposes to do, is to open up "other" places and "other" people to being included in a much larger set of questions about Western medicine, questions that address both the historical and contemporary contexts. What is the relation of the medical profession to the community, particularly when it comes to race, gender, transgender, and disability? What is the relation of medical concepts of disease to patient illness? What does the medicalized body look like from the perspective of the public, and what is the possibility of personal agency when it comes to the medicalized body? What is the relation of a market economy (hospitals, big pharma, technology) to the medical consumer? And what is the legacy of medicine in the broader arena of a medical culture?

1

## MEDICAL CULTURE

Such questions are an attempt to place medicine—that cloister of professionals that we think of as "medicine"—in the wider domain of a culture that includes patients, Dr. Moms, anatomy museums and theaters, expert testimony in the law courts, politics, the transgender community, the disability community, pharmaceutical companies and products and television drug commercials, as well as narratives about medicine from Daniel Defoe's *Journal of the Plague Year* to Margaret Edson's play *Wit*.[2] In this wider medical culture, medicine does not smell quite as sweet as it does in the traditional history of medicine. A great man like William Harvey cannot hide from the fact that his groundbreaking theory of the circulation of the blood was achieved at the expense of vivisected animals. Nor the great medical schools from the fact that their innovative pedagogy once relied on the crime of grave-robbing.

Certainly, those of us in the wider domain of medical culture have had and continue to have a conflicted relationship with medicine. It's bad enough to feel ill, but even worse to feel like a body under medical construction. Although this sense of "thing-ness" is particularly true in surgery, where doctors literally sculpt a *body* out of the *flesh*, many people experience medical treatment in general as objectifying. In fact, the public's ambivalence toward medicine has had a long history, from the horror of being dissected and publically displayed in the anatomy museum to fear of the research hospital and modern technology. Yet we still look to medicine to perform miracles. "Corrective" surgery may be dreadful to one person yet empowering to another.

Nevertheless, these comments are not intended to disrespect medicine and the superb medical advances that have been won over the course of Western history. We are living longer and better lives thanks to medicine. As a breast cancer survivor, I certainly count myself as someone who, without modern medicine, would not be treading the earth today. And as Sheena Sommers demonstrates in chapter 3 of this book, in terms of medical culture the advent of expert medical testimony in the eighteenth century was responsible for a more humane attitude shown toward women who were charged with infant murder. Yet no matter what the subject, engaging a larger cultural milieu will also show that anything "won" is not so easily won. Take the lowly medical thermometer, for example, invented in the early 1600s by Santorio Santorio (Sanctorius).[3] It is hard to imagine a diagnostic tool more elegant in its power and simplicity than the thermometer. With the thermometer, physicians were able to determine sickness based on a quantitative measure of deviation from normal body temperature. At the same time, though, the thermometer is part and parcel of a scientific culture that introduced the notion of (ab)normality into the Western world. Today, "normality" is a very uneasy notion, as Linda Seidel, following queer theorist Lennard J. Davis, argues in chapter 11 of this book.[4]

Susan Sontag was one of the first cultural writers to place medicine within the wider arena of a medical culture. As a cancer patient, she was able to have a perspective on medicine from a very important subject position: someone afflicted with a serious disease. This subject position, together with her professional training in cultural and literary studies, produced the 1978 book, *Illness as Metaphor*, in which she examined the figurative language surrounding the diseases of tuberculosis and cancer. Cancer, for instance, bears the metaphors of warfare: "[W]ith the patient's body considered to be *under attack* ("*invasion*"), the only treatment is *counterattack*" (my emphasis).[5] Such metaphors belong to medical culture, not to medicine *per se*, for they are part of the lay discourse used by, and for, nonprofessionals to talk about disease.

Some twenty years later, the Pulitzer prize-winning playwright Margaret Edson approached a similar project by looking at the professional discourse of medicine itself. Like Sontag, Edson held a subject position within medical culture, but in her case as a nonmedical clerk on the cancer and AIDS wards of a research hospital. Her play *Wit* (1999) situates an English professor, who is dying of ovarian cancer, within the domain of such a medical venue, thereby in turn generating the larger medical culture to which patients also belong. In the course of the play, the Vivian character lets loose with a literary analysis of professional medical terminology, exposing the metaphorical reverberations locked deep within such terms as "insidious." For instance, to Vivian's doctor, the word "insidious" denotes a lesion that is not detectable at an early stage of disease. To Vivian, it signifies the body's treachery.[6]

Edson and Sontag are two examples gleaned from an impressive list of historians, art historians, literary critics, body theorists, artists, and writers, as well as those medical professionals who have been thinking about the larger picture of medical culture. Undoubtedly, Michel Foucault has been one of the most influential theorists and historians, particularly in his book, *The Birth of the Clinic*, where he charts the epistemic change led by the French clinic on lesion-based medicine in the nineteenth century, which placed the body in the domain of a disease topography. Here, I want to represent the scholarly field of medical culture by mentioning a few of its developers, knowing that I leave out a great many important contributors. In the area of cultural studies: Jonathan Sawday, whose book *The Body Emblazoned* examines literary and artistic representations of Renaissance anatomy; Tim Marshall on the intersection of England's Anatomy Act and the novel *Frankenstein* in *Murdering to Dissect*; Michael Sappol on the anatomized body in nineteenth-century America in *A Traffic of Dead Bodies*; and in the twentieth and twentieth-first centuries, Elaine Scarry on physical suffering in *The Body in Pain*, Susan Bordo on anorexia in *Unbearable Weight*, and Ann Folwell Stanford on the medicalized body in novels by women of color in *Bodies in a Broken World*.

In the fine art, anatomy has played a key role in representations of the human body since the Renaissance. It is well-documented that Michelangelo and Leonardo da Vinci engaged in human dissection for the purpose of representing the human figure realistically in a wide variety of situations. Other artists have depicted medical culture itself, such as Rembrandt in *The Anatomy Lecture of Dr. Nicolaes Tulp*, in which mercantile connections to medicine provide the painting's mise en scène. The celebrated Dr. Tulp is lending his fame to a select group of bourgeois gentlemen, all of whom want to be immortalized by the most celebrated painter of the time. More recently, the plastinated bodies of Gunther von Hagens's *Body Worlds* have raised a controversy over the relation of good taste to art within the context of the medicalized body. (One might argue that discussions of taste, certainly as a bourgeois concept, have no place in art.) Today, artwork depicting medical culture may suggest, more often than not, a critical view of medicine, as is the case with Peter Greenaway's 1997 installation, *Flying over Water*, which includes a section entitled "The Autopsy Room." Here, empirical medicine is ironically juxtaposed with the myth of Icarus.

A number of physicians such as Robert April, Drew Leder, and Jacalyn Duffin have also engaged medicine as a cultural phenomenon. Theirs is a subject position that is extraordinarily valuable to students of medical culture, for they, of course, have the view from the inside of medicine. In a collection of essays that I edited, *Images of the Corpse from the Renaissance to Cyberspace*, neurologist April discusses disease concepts in postrevolutionary France as represented in the novels of Flaubert and Balzac. Leder draws on his training as a medical doctor to confront the nonexperiential body in *The Absent Body*. A physician and professor at Queen's University as well as author of *History of Medicine: A Scandalously Short Introduction*, Duffin places the history of medicine not only within the larger history of ideas, but also within the theoretical framework of constructivism.

## CONSTRUCTIVISM

Constructivism has become an important theory in the study of the body in medical culture and in medicine itself. Though he prefers the term "frame" rather than "construct," Charles E. Rosenberg points out, in the introduction to *Framing Disease*, that a disease only comes to exist when we name it.[7] Rosenberg, as well as Duffin, expresses a general agreement among students of medical culture today that a disease belongs to the system of classification used to describe and categorize the set of symptoms that patients are experiencing.[8] As Duffin writes, illness and disease are two different terms: "The word 'illness' is used to designate individual suffering; the word 'disease,' pertains to ideas about the illness."[9]

Constructivism enables historians of medicine to think of their subject in terms of changing concepts rather than in terms of discoveries. Steven J. Peitzman offers the history of renal (kidney) disease as a case in point. Before the nineteenth century, renal disease was known as "dropsy." Dropsy had a set of symptoms, edema among them, that fit neatly into the humoral model of the body, a model that had been operative since Aristotle.[10] In the 1820s, the physician Richard Bright correlated patient symptoms to specific urine chemistry and lesions in the kidney at autopsy.[11] Renal disease was now modeled according to chemical and lesion-based pathology and renamed Bright's Disease, after its researcher. Today, renal disease is organized around dialysis and is termed "end-stage renal disease" or ESRD. ESRD is an administrative term reflective of the technology used to treat renal disease and belongs to the discourse used by medical providers and insurance payers.[12]

The history of renal disease, then, is actually a history of changing concepts and models of the body, not a history of illness. The illness experienced by patients remains the same over time, though today because of diagnostic and treatment technologies patients with ESRD mostly experience the discomfort of dialysis rather than feel sick from dropsy or Bright's Disease. In fact, one can recognize in the general history of medicine how changing ideas in philosophy and science have intersected with the practice of medicine and the understanding of the body.

Humoral medicine lasted from the ancients well into the eighteenth century and was based on the idea in natural philosophy of a balance among the four elements of the world.[13] Nevertheless, by the early Renaissance, empiricism had taken hold of the scientific community, leading not only to the teaching of anatomy in medical schools, but also to the later development of lesion-based classification. Although it presented a challenge to humoral medicine, anatomy seemed to have little value to the clinician who continued to treat patients according to the humors. Mechanistic theories introduced during the seventeenth century by philosophers such as Descartes led to the modeling of the body as a mechanical object. Such a concept was invaluable to someone like Harvey, for it enabled him to conceive of the heart as a "pump." The "new science" of Newton, with its empirical and mathematical methods, not only introduced technologies such as the microscope into medical research, it would eventually found Mendelian genetics, arguably the greatest scientific model of the body conceived to date. Throughout the twentieth and early twenty-first centuries, technology in the forms of research, diagnosis, and treatment has contributed to ever more finely tuned concepts of the body, even those like ESRD that are bureaucratically driven.

## THE BODY

So far, I have been discussing constructivism as it pertains to the construction of concepts of disease and models of the body in medicine. However, constructivism has also led to debates in body criticism circles as to whether the *body* is itself constructed. One side of the debate led by Judith Butler and followed mostly by a contingent of queer theorists argues that the body is constructed "all the way down," to borrow the conference phrase.[14] In many ways, such a viewpoint rings true especially with respect to surgery, though perhaps the term "reconstruct" better suits the situation than the term "construct." After all, the fleshy material is already there in some human form. Sex reassignment surgery, discussed by Sally Hines in chapter 9 of this book, is a clear case of reconstruction of the body, though many other medical treatments, including drug regimens, also inscribe their mark on the body and make of it a readable cultural object.

In *Bodies That Matter*, Butler's project is to deconstruct the binary of materiality and culture, particularly the way regulatory norms rigidify sex, by showing how the body is always constructed by culture and posited in language.[15] There are two problems that arise with such a project as Butler's, certainly when applied to medical culture. The first problem lies in the object of analysis. The body under examination in Butlerian analysis is a body that has been *culturally* medicalized rather than a body that is strictly a medical construct. As Rosenberg points out, such medicalized bodies cannot be proved to have an underlying "biopathological mechanism." He gives the examples of hysteria, chlorosis, neurasthenia, and homosexuality, diagnoses that are "culturally resonant."[16] Such bodies truly are nothing more than cultural objects, since they do not have a provable biomedical aspect, though the treatment can certainly affect the body. And, as we know, several of these "diseases" are no longer considered diseases in medicine.

Immediately, a second problem arises in considering what happens to the body when the analysis of a culturally medicalized body is transferred to the materiality/culture binary. In taking the binary apart, the materiality of the body (the fleshy stuff) ends up going under erasure, while the cultural body is left looming large. Cultural constructivism takes over the body "all the way down." The other side of the debate, then, would want to preserve the materiality, the reality, indeed the fleshy stuff of the body. Certainly, in the reality of medical culture, we know that the flesh cannot be "erased," however much we would like it to go away. People become ill, people die regardless of the cultural constructs of medicine—the research, the diagnoses, the treatments.

It seems to me that a better way of thinking through the binary, if it is indeed a binary, of materiality and culture, lies in the realm of the dialectic. Rather than a zero-sum game (no matter-all culture), the two sides can be recognized as mutually in play. Terry Eagleton and Kate Soper develop this dialectic in their respective books, *The Idea of Culture* and *What is Nature?* Eagleton uses the example of poverty. Poor people have larger than normal adrenal glands due to stress, "but poverty is not able to create adrenal glands where none exist."[17] Though Soper is discussing the dialectic of nature and culture, her viewpoint enables one to see a place for the materiality of the body, which belongs to the realm of nature, outside of the purview of cultural constructs without putting the body under erasure: Certain materialities fall outside the product of human activity, and, in fact, "are the necessary condition of every human practice, and determine the possible forms it can take."[18] In terms of a dialectic regarding materiality and culture, one can say that the material body exerts conditions on the shape(s) of cultural constructs, and at the same time the cultural constructs inflect the flesh.

Such a dialectic rests on what I have called elsewhere *constructivist realism*.[19] Constructivist realism relies on the philosophical theory of realism, which states in its simplest form that an external reality exists outside of cultural representation.[20] Yet constructivist realism also concedes the reality of humanly built structures, whether those structures are in the form of bridges and roads, the conceptual models of medicine, or the medicalized body. This term is useful, I think, in enabling us to recognize a place for the body's materiality beyond culture, but at the same time to understand a dialectic of play between materiality and culture. At their base, the chapters in this book accept the existence of the material flesh and consider it to be distinct from the medicalized body. That said, they focus on the ways in which the *body* is constructed within the wider context of medical culture—expert medical testimony, the drug advertisement, the anatomy museum, and so on.

## THE BODY IN MEDICAL CULTURE

I have chosen the chapters for *The Body in Medical Culture* in the spirit of cultural studies. Not only is the body perceived as an artifact in medical culture, but the book also displays how scholars working in cultural studies approach this topic, specifically the negotiation of medical models and constructions of the body in the community at large, whether the community is high, low or middle brow, or finds itself in the venues of elite culture, the Internet, or television. The book reflects a wide range of topics, including early modern medical manuals, anatomy museums and blackface minstrelsy, biomedical ethics, drugs such as Vioxx, disability, the patient "object" of doctor jokes, medical transgendering, and designer vaginas, among others. Moreover, the authors approach the subject from various methodologies within the interdisciplines of cultural studies: For instance, Sally Hines and co-authors Lisa Gabbert and Antonio Salud II take a sociological approach in analyzing empirical data, while Hillary Nunn and Stephen Johnson examine primary material from the British Library, the Folger Shakespeare Library, and the Wellcome Library for the History of Medicine. And the authors represent a wide range of disciplines: medicine, women's studies, comparative literature, English, American literature, American studies, folklore, creative writing, sociology, drama studies, and history.

Though the book is organized according to an historical time line, it is not meant to be taken as a seamless history. Rather, each chapter operates as a snapshot of some moment in medical culture, whether eighteenth-century expert medical testimony or twenty-first-century digital anatomy. "Home Bodies: Matters of Weight in Renaissance Women's Medical Manuals," is concerned with the manuscripts of home recipe books, written in large part by women, that were gleaned by Hillary M. Nunn from the archives of the Folger Shakespeare Library and the Wellcome Library. Nunn analyzes these manuals for their interest in body size and weight in early modern English culture, showing how food was not merely a matter of taste or maintaining humoral balance, but also a way of constructing the body through prescriptive home medicine, "to make a greate body small."[21] Moreover, in correcting a scholarly tradition that has tended to see medicine in the Renaissance as the sole purview of (male) physicians, anatomists, and barber surgeons, Nunn brings to our attention the important role played by early modern women, in tending to the health of their families and tenants, as cultural arbiters of body size and health.

Nevertheless, the authority lay women have had in medical culture since the Renaissance has always ended up yielding to the jurisdiction of the professional physician. During the eighteenth century, physicians, who were authorized to perform autopsies, began to replace midwives as the experts not only in determining cause of death in unattended births, but also in evaluating the accused mother's state of mind. The corpse of the

infant became the empirical site through which culpability on the part of
the mother would be determined, and thus the construction of a readable
infant corpse was a precondition to constructing the functioning of an
accused woman's mind. Sheena Sommers examined more than 180 Old
Bailey proceedings on infant murder during the eighteenth century to
write chapter 2, "Remapping Maternity in the Courtroom: Female
Defenses and Medical Witnesses in Eighteenth-Century Infanticide
Proceedings." In a surprising twist, Sommers discovered that the conviction rates for women charged with infanticide declined with the onset of
expert medical testimony.

The construction of the dead body plays a significant role as well in
chapter 3 by Stephen Johnson, which explores the relationship between the
skeleton in the anatomical museum and the blackface minstrel on the variety stage, both popular images in mid-nineteenth-century United States and
Britain. Despite evoking the extremes of complete control or wild abandon,
Johnson reads these seemingly disparate forms as deploying a common
theme: the body aggressively manipulated either through the denuding of
flesh or a cultural "blackening up." In particular, Johnson examines the
case of William (Juba) Lane, the only performer of color on the segregated
minstrel stage during its early years (the 1840s), whose skeleton was purportedly on display in the anatomy museum shortly after his death while
touring Britain in 1852. "'Surely he cannot be flesh and blood': The Early
Victorian Anatomical Museum and the Blackface Minstrel" draws extensively on documentary evidence from the British Library, the Wellcome
Library, local archives, and nineteenth-century periodicals.

While Johnson writes of racial issues and the medicalization of the
black body, Hayley Mitchell Haugen explores gender and the fabrication of
the disabled masculine body in the early to mid-twentieth century when
polio epidemics were sweeping the land and shattering the bodies and
dreams of many children. At a time when American manhood was already
being questioned, disability was especially acute for boys who found themselves "emasculated" by the disease and stigmatized as "cripples."
Ironically, though perhaps not surprisingly, the very images of masculinity
torn from the disabled patient returned to haunt the discourse of medical
culture, rendered in expressions such as "beating polio like a man." In this
chapter, "The 'Disabled Imagination' and the Masculine Metaphor in the
Works of Leonard Kriegel," Haugen looks specifically at the autobiographical writings of one man who, disabled by polio at the age of eleven, relied
on intensive weight training to sculpt a masculine body and, thus, to construct a "heroic self."

What happens when the fabric of the body is broken is a topic also
considered by Catalina Florina Florescu in chapter 5, "Of Genes,

Mutations, and Desires in Franz Kafka's *The Metamorphosis* and Moacyr Scliar's *The Centaur in the Garden*." Drawing on Drew Leder's definition in *The Absent Body* of "dys-appearance" as a bodily state potentially initiated by a diagnosis of terminal illness, Florescu reads these works as examples of a "body-broken" undergoing mutation.[22] When the flesh has been broken, whether by illness or some unexplained cause, these narratives create a space in which to embody the animal contained in the civilized human construct or vice versa. Florescu shows that the animal phase, as bug or centaur, is terrifying, in large part because combining human tissue with an animal counterpart is a project of hybridity and, thus, brings with it a host of alarming ethical questions.

Similar ethical questions are broached in the next chapter by Natalia Lizama. Lizama addresses the "mutation" of two human beings into their digital counterparts, specifically the Visible Human Project (VHP) funded by the National Library of Medicine and one of its spin-off CD programs, *BodyVoyage* by Alexander Tsiaras. In the mid-1990s, researchers sectioned a male and a female cadaver into thin slices, photographed the planar edges, and uploaded the information into a database that could be used for pedagogical or artistic purposes. Though on the one hand, the VHP may be an honorable effort in the enlightenment tradition, Lizama argues that the digital fabrication of the human being has, perhaps unwittingly, produced a "post-biological affect" of two distinct kinds: post-biological horror and post-biological nostalgia. In chapter 6, "The Post-biological Body: Horror, Nostalgia, and the Visible Human Project," Lizama shows that in an age of posthumanist, digital anatomy, the "authentic" anatomical body may be neither particularly natural nor authentic.

Access to the interior of the body is problematic as well to Catherine Belling in chapter 7, "Endography: A Physician's Dream of Omniscience." She analyzes the novels of Robin Cook, a physician-turned-writer, for their "endography," a term Belling coins to describe the "physician-novelist's effort to construct and convey an impossible omniscient access" to the live body's interior.[23] Like Lizama in the previous chapter, Belling questions the belief that medical technology provides access to the inside of the body: If the body is live, that access is profoundly limited by the mediation of imaging machines or by the constraints of surgery; if the body is dead, that access is limited by, well, deadness. In Cook's novels, Belling sees an interdisciplinary attempt to combine clinical medicine with suspense fiction in order to fashion, through language, a bodily interior that can be both alive and accessible. She also sees, though, that Cook's particular focus on female bodies, whether as protagonists or victims—what she terms "gynopsy"—demonstrates a discomforting alliance of medical knowledge and power.

A related form of "gynopsy" is under discussion in Alexa A. Priddy and Jennifer L. Croissant's essay "Designer Vaginas," which explores the reconstructed vagina as the latest fashion in cosmetic surgery. Though some vaginal surgeries are conducted for health reasons, most are performed to force an "unruly" vagina into a more culturally normative appearance. As with other body projects in the United States, Priddy and Croissant argue that the designer vagina invokes a dilemma not only for individual women but also for feminists by raising the question of cultural control of the female body on the one hand and personal agency on the other. Toward the end of the essay, Priddy and Croissant rightly compare the designer vagina to "female genital mutilation" in Africa. Though they are remarkably similar procedures (and done for similar reasons), U.S. discourse on female genital mutilation reveals a cultural bias against Africa, for African women are seen as having less agency than their American counterparts.

If the discourse on the designer vagina is centered on the idea of having the "wrong vagina," Sally Hines shows that discourse on transgender is similarly yoked to the idea of having the "wrong body." In chapter 9, "(Trans) Gendered Fabrication and the Surgery Debates," Hines reports the conclusions of a research project in which she interviewed thirty transgendered men and women to investigate how sex-change surgery is viewed by this community. She not only questions the narrative of the "wrong body," initiated by medical discourse and now rampant in the transgender community, but also questions the benefit of surgical procedures "to correct" it. As with the designer vagina, reconstructive surgery is a permanent, nontrivial resculpting of the flesh in order to produce a seemingly more "natural," "natural-appearing," or "true" body. Hines discovered in the course of conducting this research that the surgically reconstructed body is a topic of heated debate in the transgender community.

Similarly, in the next chapter, Lisa Gabbert and Antonio Salud II examine the so-called natural body in the venue of the hospital. The modern hospital routinely disciplines the unruly flesh by regulating its functions through sleep, food, and dress regimens, activity, social space, and so on. Gabbert and Salud have also discovered, though, a subversive discourse at work in the hospital where off-color body jokes are directed by medical personnel against patients, diseases, procedures, and other staff members. To explain this contradictory aspect of medical culture, the authors define the body as a contested site of meaning, ideology, and social reality, with the "medical carnivalesque" mediating a medical venue that is both in- and out-of-control, disciplinary and humanitarian. Chapter 10, "On Slanderous Words and Bodies-Out-of-Control: Hospital Humor and the Medical Carnivalesque," draws on ethnographic research as well as literary renderings, the media, and collections of hospital folklore to analyze "doctor jokes."

The foregoing chapters tend to focus on a body in medical culture that each of us may or may not be able personally to identify with, depending, of course, not only on historical time period, but also on our individual gender, race, degree of ableness or sickness, and so on. However, the concluding chapter by Linda Seidel is about a body all of us know or soon will: the aging body. In chapter 11, "Dr. Jarvik and Other Baby Boomers: (Still) Performing the Able Body," Seidel shows how the marketing of drugs, supplements and surgeries on television targets a middle-aged and older audience by convincing us that "normal" means "youthful." Viewers are pressured into medicalizing their own bodies by badgering their doctors into prescribing drugs and other regimens that are designed to construct a body more suitable to a market economy. The chapter ends by suggesting that such advertising also publicizes the fact that we are all in the same boat, and that we could, ironically, decide to support each other in resisting the compulsory youthful body.

Indeed, Seidel's activist position brings to a point a motif running through all the chapters in this book: Despite the insistence of the flesh, the *body* in medical culture can never be claimed as true, natural, or normal, whether Renaissance women are managing its weight or disabled men are sculpting its muscles. Nevertheless, the more thought we give to the ways in which the body has been, and continues to be, fabricated in Western culture, the more likely we are to have a positive finale: The body in medical culture may actually be a body open to personal agency, even political agency, if we have the desire to construct it.

## NOTES

1. Michael Neve, "Conclusion," *The Western Medical Tradition*, the Wellcome Institute for the History of Medicine (London: Cambridge University Press, 1995), 478.

2. I am using the term "medical culture" somewhat differently than Deborah Lupton's use of the term "medicine as culture" in her book *Medicine as Culture*. Lupton's book focuses on the medical profession in a context informed by various theories of culture drawn from a number of disciplines—sociology, feminism, anthropology, and so on. See Deborah Lupton, *Medicine as Culture: Illness, Disease, and the Body in Western Societies* (London: Sage, 1994). To my mind, "medical culture" strikes an anthropological chord, where the term indicates a community broader than the medical profession. In fact, Catherine Belling tells me that U.S. culture itself should be considered a "medical culture."

3. Andrew Wear, "Medicine in Early Modern Europe, 1500-1700," *The Western Medical Tradition*, the Wellcome Institute for the History of Medicine (London: Cambridge University Press, 1995), 354.

4. Linda Seidel, "Dr. Jarvik and Other Baby Boomers: (Still) Performing the Able Body," *The Body in Medical Culture*, ed. Elizabeth Klaver (Albany: SUNY Press, 2009) 229-241. See also Lennard J. Davis, *Bending over Backwards: Disability, Dismodernism, and Other Difficult Positions* (New York: New York UP, 2002) and Michael Warner, *The Trouble with Normal: Sex, Politics, and the Ethics of Queer Life* (Cambridge: Harvard UP, 1999).

5. Susan Sontag, *Illness as Metaphor and Aids and Its Metaphors* (New York: Picador, 2001), 64.

6. Margaret Edson, *Wit* (New York: Dramatists Play Service, 1999), 9.

7. Charles E. Rosenberg, Introduction, "Framing Disease: Illness, Society, and History," *Framing Disease*, ed. Charles E. Rosenberg and Janet Golden (New Brunswick: Rutgers University Press, 1992), xiii.

8. Ibid., xv.

9. Jacalyn Duffin, *History of Medicine: A Scandalously Short Introduction* (Toronto: University of Toronto Press, 1999), 66.

10. Steven J. Peitzman, "From Bright's Disease to End-Stage Renal Disease," in *Framing Disease*, ed. Charles E. Rosenberg and Janet Golden (New Brunswick: Rutgers University Press, 1992), 3.

11. Ibid., 9.

12. Ibid., 14.

13. Wear, "Medicine in Early Modern Europe," 360, 261-62.

14. According to Butler, the very stuff that makes up the world, including the body, is constructed. For instance, she defines matter as "*a process of materialization that stabilizes over time to produce the effect of boundary, fixity, and surface we call matter*" (9). This definition ends up trapping matter in a discursive loop. Judith Butler, *Bodies That Matter: On the Discursive Limits of Sex* (New York: Routledge, 1993), 9. Terry Eagleton critiques a similar phrase: "If culture really does go *all the way down*, then it seems to play just the same role as nature" (my emphasis). *The Idea of Culture* (Oxford: Blackwell, 2000), 94.

15. Butler, see Introduction, *Bodies That Matter*, 1-12.

16. Rosenberg, "Introduction," xv.

17. Eagleton, *The Idea of Culture*, 87.

18. Kate Soper, *What is Nature? Culture, Politics, and the Non-Human* (Oxford: Blackwell, 1995), 132-33.

19. Elizabeth Klaver, *Sites of Autopsy in Contemporary Culture* (Albany: SUNY Press, 2005), 43-56.

20. John Searle, *The Construction of Social Reality* (New York: The Free Press, 1995), 155.

21. Hillary M. Nunn, "Home Bodies: Matters of Weight in Renaissance Women's Medical Manuals," *The Body in Medical Culture*, ed. Elizabeth Klaver (Albany: SUNY Press 2009) 15–36.

22. Drew Leder, *The Absent Body* (Chicago : University of Chicago Press, 1990), 84, quoted in Catalina Florina Florescu, "Of Genes, Mutations, and Desires in Kafka, Scliar, and Schultz," *The Body in Medical Culture*, ed. Elizabeth Klaver (Albany: SUNY Press 2009) 109–124.

23. Catherine Belling, "Endography: A Physician's Dream of Omniscience," *The Body in Medical Culture*, ed. Elizabeth Klaver (Albany: SUNY Press 2009) 151–172.

ONE

# Home Bodies

## *Matters of Weight in Renaissance Women's Medical Manuals*

HILLARY M. NUNN

ONE OF THE MOST ENDURING images of the English Renaissance is that of King Henry VIII, often imagined in terms of his appetites, firmly planted at a banquet table with a turkey leg in his hand. In modern-day popular culture, he is pictured as a gruff, commandeering gourmand, even a glutton, whose eating constitutes an integral component of his public and private identity.[1] At the same time, this image of Henry works to reinforce the modern notion that body size was not seen as medically significant in his times. If anything, today's popular views of the Renaissance emphasize that Henry-like heft served as a cultural indication of privilege, revealing his access to substantial quantities of food, and that what today would be seen as obesity once constituted a sign of high financial and cultural status. Yet most Renaissance medical authorities on diet—and everyday observers, for that matter—did not endorse the indulgent eating or girth so often associated with today's image of King Henry. In fact, even Henry's contemporaries commented on the effects his voracious eating had on his behavior and physical condition, and, in the king's later years, onlookers labeled his size as a factor in his declining health.[2]

As such comments make clear, popular and learned Renaissance notions of the body's inner functions made food choices much more than

15

reflections of preference and privilege, and neither obesity nor extreme thinness met with the approval of those involved in health care. Instead, the era's overarching concern with inner humoral balance, rooted in the ancient traditions of Greek medicine in the time of Galen, transformed the question of what to eat into a medical issue.[3] While experimental medicine gradually began to erode the dominance of the Galenic model among elite scientists as the seventeenth century progressed, the centuries-old notion of the humors held firm in popular circles. As Ken Albala argues in his study of printed Renaissance discussions of eating, the era's experts envisioned the foods an individual ingested as exercising immediate effects on his internal workings, altering the proportions of blood, phlegm, choler, and bile that interacted within the body. Because each person's body existed as a unique combination of these humors, every dish on a menu would cause a different internal reaction for each diner at a given table, affecting individual digestive systems in markedly different ways. As a result, the largely female task of food preparation became, in Albala's words, "a matter not only of rendering foods more palatable and digestible but of counteracting food's adverse qualities by balancing them with correcting condiments."[4]

While male authors of printed books dealt almost exclusively with explaining the theory behind digestion, it fell to women to deal with the practical challenges of feeding and nursing the members of their households. Furthermore, most early modern households had little access to the sorts of university-trained doctors whose published work is most available to those today who study Renaissance health care.[5] These books, too, were rare and prohibitively expensive in their time, and the texts' specialized vocabularies catered to readers with a far greater level of literacy than that enjoyed by the typical English woman.[6] Renaissance women could turn to printed household manuals, generally written by men, yet these too proved expensive and often took a didactic tone.[7] Instead, women frequently turned to a remarkable, but often overlooked, variety of health-care literature. Women, and often men, created their own handwritten medical manuals, sometimes called receipt books, for use in their homes. These books were more than just notebooks of random recipes; they were typically well-organized, sturdily bound volumes that recorded procedures for treating medical problems along with instructions for making a wide variety of chemical and herbal treatments.[8] The household manuscripts that many women consulted—and wrote—mingled cookery and medicinal recipes, thus exemplifying the era's penchant for blending concerns regarding eating and health care.

Manuscript books of cookery recipes and home remedies serve as reflections of the everyday practice of medical care during the late sixteenth and early seventeenth centuries. Household manuals dating before the Restoration—my main concern in this chapter—show a striking awareness not just of food's role in maintaining the body's inner balance, but of the effect that eating's most visible result—body size—could have on the individual's overall health. Though Renaissance interest in weight control has long been overlooked, these manuscripts demonstrate a striking understanding of the importance of body size as a medical issue, devoting space to food-based cures "to make a great body small" and to aid those suffering from an "appetite lost."[9] Such home medical manuals assign a significant role to appetite and body size in individual health. Just as importantly, these books forge for female readers and authors powerful cultural positions as arbiters of eating—and as knowledgeable medical practitioners—not just in the early modern household but in Renaissance culture at large.

## WOMEN WRITERS, BODY SIZE, AND HOUSEHOLD MEDICAL MANUSCRIPTS

For years, scholars have claimed that people in the early modern period showed no concern regarding their weight, and, strictly speaking, that may well be so. Albala, for example, states that none of the era's many diet regimens "was designed to help the reader lose weight, and rarely was body size a major concern, except that the average or mean size was considered most healthy"; he grants, however, that medical writers after 1570 emphasize that "body size should be corrected," with fat people eating "thinning foods" and thin people eating "fattening foods."[10] This preference for a healthy, unspecified medium body size is certainly assumed in the era's home medical manuals, yet to state that these collections of advice and home remedies show no interest in matters of bodily girth, or lack thereof, is overstating the case. True, treatments in household manuscripts usually make no reference to a patient's measured weight; however, home medical books commonly contain recipes designed to alter the bodies and influence the appetites of their patients, thereby indicating that concerns for physical size, wrapped up in the modern term "weight," constituted a legitimate early modern health issue.

English women typically took charge of their families' meals and health, and gentlewomen who lived on country estates often saw it as their duty to tend to the health of those who lived within the bounds of their manors. While visiting London, Emanuel Van Meteren remarked that women enjoyed "the free management of the house" and, though they preferred to leave most work to their servants, ventured "to market to buy what they like best to eat."[11] Such observations of the privileged city woman's public life necessarily obscure even as they enlighten, for they use women's activities outside of the house to speculate on her activities within it. Even so, Van Meteren's comment offers us a glimpse at the control city women had over food consumption in their households. While they may not have cooked the meals or prepared medicines themselves, women oversaw the activities of their usually female kitchen servants.[12] At the same time, sixteenth- and seventeenth-century London's medical marketplace began to undergo substantial changes, as university-educated medical practitioners sought increased power to regulate those who made their livings caring for the sick. The results of these efforts, however, need not have altered the ways that a woman saw to her family's health, especially in the countryside. Medical doctors, after all, were in short supply in these areas, and their services were priced well beyond what most inhabitants of the provinces could afford. While rural women who provided care typically underwent no formal medical education, they learned from those around them and in some cases from their reading; the more aristocratic among them may also have been influenced by traditional notions of their responsibility to the communities surrounding their estates.[13] The close connections between preparing food and medicines—which, after all, were often made of the same ingredients—made the medicinal work these women undertook a seemingly natural fit.

The household manuals that these Renaissance Englishwomen consulted were themselves an eclectic assortment of advice and recipes that would today be variously classified as cookbooks, chemistry texts, first-aid manuals, and home health-care guides. The era's cookery manuscripts include a bewildering variety of recipes for preparing food and medicine—and these categories often overlap. For example, Lady Anne Fettiplace's 225-page household book, dating from 1604, contains more than three hundred medical recipes, including fifty-six for dressing wounds and two dozen cures to comfort the stomach.[14] Not only did women prepare most of the household compounds used in health care, cleaning, and food preservation; they had a limited number of ingredients on hand from which to make these important products. Many recipes look alike simply because they rely on native plants and other on-hand materials rather than exotic commodities that could be obtained through trade. While medical and culinary preparations often involved the same ingredients, these manuscripts usually attempt to separate the two different varieties of recipes, giving each category its own place within the book. Yet those distinctions do not prove firm, as medical recipes often pop up on unexpected pages among the foodstuffs, and the alphabetical arrangement of some texts seemingly ignores the supposed division between products to be eaten for sustenance and those to be ingested as medicine.

While manuscript, and sometimes printed, recipe books usually constituted a housewife's main source of medical information, some household libraries provided women with the comparative luxury of printed medical handbooks, written by university-trained physicians or, more often, by less educated practitioners who hoped to offer basic medical instruction to those in need. In addition, many homes contained a copy of an herbal, a book describing local plants and their medicinal uses. Lady Margaret Hoby's diary, for example, suggests she had both kinds of books at her disposal; she makes reference to reading an herbal and to reading Timothy Bright's A treatise on melancholy as well.[15] Her voracious reading—not just of medical books but of her Bible—makes Hoby a remarkably literate woman for her day, and her diary underscores her position as a producer as well as consumer of literary materials; she keeps careful records of her visits to the sick and her treatment of the injured, often happily reporting her successes.

Most women in the country, however, seemed to rely on manuscript books passed from generation to generation within their families. For example, Fettiplace's recipe book passed first to her niece and then back into her direct family line during the eighteenth century; the book continues to be passed among members of her extended family today.[16] Rebecca Brandreth, meanwhile, bequeathed two such household volumes to her daughter Anne in 1740.[17] As Sara Pennell notes, however, the authorship of household manuscripts is not always clear-cut. Recipe books attributed to women often reveal traces of male scribal penmanship, and some men appear to have actively added to their families' medical handbooks as well.[18] Despite such male involvement, Pennell maintains not only that these books link women to medical duties, but that such manuals allow women to connect with one another across generations.

These manuscripts often record standard recipes for curing common illnesses, sometimes offering clues to a recipe's origin. Notes in the margins of some books reveal that writers often copied recipes from borrowed texts, or that particular doctors or neighbors offered individual recorded prescriptions.[19] In most cases, however, the manuscripts offer few clues as to whether their medical cures describe local customs for treatment, or perhaps medical recipes derived by an individual author. While manuscript owners occasionally make notes about a particular recipe's origin, most cures have little in the way of explanation or history attached to them. Whatever the recipe's history, the household manuscripts make clear that these medical treatments often underwent some degree of revision. In use for centuries in some cases, these books contain the handwriting of mothers, daughters, and sometimes granddaughters, with later users adding their own recipes and modifying those that earlier writers had recorded and even constructing indexes and tables of contents to make consulting the book simpler for future users.[20]

## TREATING THE APPETITES

The era's household manuscripts vividly illustrate the extent to which medicine and eating were intertwined. While some recipes later in the early modern period offer extensive detail regarding the steps involved in preparing foods and medicines, many offer few particulars as to measurements and procedures.[21] Recipes dealing with treatments for discomforts relating to food and appetite illustrate the brevity frequently exhibited in the form. For example, Katherine Packer's 1639 manuscript names wormwood as a prescription to "purge the stomach from all grossness," but does not specify how much of the herb should be used or even how it should be administered.[22] Such instructions hint that many medical manuscripts served primarily as prompts, jolting the users' memory to recall a simple, familiar household approach to treating a particular condition. While Elizabeth Tebeaux argues that, by the seventeenth century, printed household manuals had developed their own brand of technical writing, it is clear that their manuscript counterparts still frequently functioned as simple mnemonic devices, offering only lists of ingredients, as Packer's seventeenth-century book illustrates.[23] Other manuscripts, however, offer more detail in their preparations. The Stanhope family receipt book, for example, describes the following procedures: "To make one fat, in a short time": "Take new milk from the cow and fair running water of each a like quantity, sweeten it with sugar candy, and drink every morning fasting, and a good draught thereof."[24] The recipe provides no precise measurements, but it does offer specifics of when and how the cure should be administered.

Another manuscript typical of the genre, compiled between 1625 and 1700 by an unknown author, offers an elaborately brewed concoction to comfort a wide array of health issues and even to serve as a preventative medicine. The recipe's seemingly outlandish mélange of snails, earthworms, and herbs purports to cure a range of apparently contradictory symptoms, ranging from surfeit—a condition we would call indigestion, usually linked to overeating—to loss of appetite. Taken habitually, the author claims that the concoction aids in maintaining good digestion. First, the author instructs, the housewife should wash a peck of garden snails and put them on the fire, then let them rest [in the fire] till they have done making a noise, then take them forth, and with a knife and coarse cloth pick and wipe them from the ashes, coals, and green froth yet is in them, then bruise them[,] shells and all[,] in a stone mortar [;] take also a quart of earth worms, slit and scour them with salt, then wash them well from their filth, and beat them well in a stone mortar…[then combine] 2 handfuls of Angelica, and as many Celandine upon that, then put in 2. quarts of rosemary flowers, Bearsfoot, Agrimony, the reddest dock roots, the bark of Barberries tree wood sorrel, and Betony of each 2 handful, of Rue, half a handful, fenugreek and Turmeric well beaten of each an ounce, then lay your snails and worms on the top of your herbs and flowers, then put in three gallons of the strongest Ale, and so let it stand all night or longer in the place where you make your fire under it[;] then in the morning put in 3 ounces of cloves beaten to powder, [six ounces grated hartshorn and] six penny weight of saffron beaten to a powder.…

The recipe concludes with advice that sounds surprisingly modern, telling practitioners to "take of this water 2. spoonfuls in a morning with 4 spoonful of beer, and the like proportion at four of the clock in the afternoon" before advising that patients should "other wise use good diet and moderate exercise to warm the blood."[25]

As the above recipe hints, the same ingredients could be used to treat the seemingly contradictory symptoms of overeating and lost appetite. According to early modern theories of digestion, however, both conditions ultimately stem from a loss of heat in the body, resulting in a "cold stomach"—that is, one that cannot generate adequate warmth to digest food. Such a loss of internal heat could make a patient lose all desire to eat, while, at the other extreme, eating too much could smother the internal fire needed to move food through the digestive system. In either case, the suffering person needed a medicine to rekindle his/her digestive processes. Hence, a Folger Shakespeare Library copy of John Partridge's printed *Treasurie of commodious conceits*, once owned by a woman named Catherine Tallemache, recommends oil of wormwood both to cure surfeit and stimulate hunger: "It is hot, and comforteth the parts that are too much cooled, chiefly the stomach, provoketh appetite, taketh away obstructions, and killeth worms."[26]

Both manuscript and printed sources contain a wide variety of recipes designed to relieve the symptoms of surfeit. These formulas typically involve diuretic herbal blends, and many multiuse medicinal waters claim relief of surfeit as one of their properties. The manuscript collection that offers the medicinal use of snails described above, for example, includes a recipe for a cordial water to treat "any infectious disease, or the plague, pox, measles, or pestilent burning fever, or to remove any offensive or venomous matter from the heart or stomach, or to be used after a surfeit, or in passions of the mother, or for children in fits of convulsions."[27] The promise of relief from indigestion among these discomforts is hardly surprising, since the list is populated by ailments that would require the body to be purged of offending agents, whether they be the plague or unconcoctible food. Not all recipes, however, relied on that sort of logic. For example, Katherine Packer's manuscript remedy collection simply orders the patient suffering from surfeit to "eat as much fine white hard sugar as a walnut."[28] Other recipes promising relief included mixtures of raisins with brandy, herbs and malmsey,[29] and poppies in conjunction with raisins or figs.[30]

Even more common were recipes claiming to stimulate appetite. Unlike most formulas for curing surfeit, recipes for provoking appetite in the healthy often involved preparations that could pass for courses in a meal rather than medicinal preparations. Albala points out that printed medicinal books took to prescribing lettuce salads before meals to calm the stomach and prepare it for better digestive functioning.[31] The prescriptions for less healthy patients who could or would not eat, however, prove less appetizing. As usual, the recipes offer little advice about when such medicines should be administered, so it is difficult to know whether they were designed for otherwise healthy patients who simply could not or would not eat, or patients suffering from other diseases that made eating difficult. Jane Jackson's recipe book contains a tonic especially designed to bring hunger back to those suffering from "humours coming to the mouth of the stomach"; the same collection also recommends centaury plant "for a man that hath no stomach to his meat."[32] Another manuscript medical miscellany provides a recipe for a "broth to keep one from wasting."[33] Packer's book offers an all-purpose vinegar concoction designed to open up internal blockages that might hinder the body's health and appetite. Labeled a recipe "To make syrup of vinegar for the stopping in the stomach & to voice phlegm & to procure appetite to meat," Packer's recipe is atypically specific regarding the medicine's production and administration:

> Take half a p[in]t of wine vinegar & half a p[in]t of running water & boil in it a handful unset slop & a sprig of red fennel & when it is half boiled away then pour it from the herbs into a pewter dish & boil it with fine sugar on a chafing dish & coals until it be a syrup[.] [T]ake a spoonful morning & evening or at any time.[34]

Packer's recipe combines fennel, an herb that we shall see is often recommended for slimming purposes, with the diuretic vinegar to purge the patient's body, theoretically voiding all the internal blockages that create a lack of appetite.

For most healthy people, moderation was the watchword as far as eating and food choice were concerned, and the era's letters and diaries show a keen awareness of the link between overindulgence and the pain of surfeit. For example, Lady Anne Clifford's diary entries connect her overindulgence in fruits and cheese to short-term illnesses.[35] Katherine Paston, meanwhile, urges her son at university to be careful in his eating. She begins her letter dated March of 1625 with her happiness at hearing of her son's good health, adding that she hopes "so long as thou be every way moderate in thy recreations and careful and temperate in thy diet... it will still increase." Echoing the tone of modern mothers warning their college-bound sons of the hazards of an all-pizza diet, Paston then warns of the particular evils of

> those possetty curdy drinks which howsoever pleasing to the pallet it maybe for a time, yet I am persuaded are most unwholesome and very Clogging to the stomach and apt to breed surfeits by reason they do not readily digest but many times do corrupt in the stomach....[36]

Paston's motherly medical advice cautions against overindulgence, warning her son about the damage his bad habits could bring to his health; moreover, her insistence reflects not just the era's humoral theories of inner bodily workings but its perceptions of the dangerous results of clogging the digestion with too much, or the wrong kinds of, food.

## BODY SIZE IN HOUSEHOLD MEDICAL TREATMENTS

Popular culture reflected the notion that overindulgence in food could cause both long and short-term harm to a person's physical makeup. Despite the jovial figures cut by rotund characters like Shakespeare's Falstaff and the real-life poet Ben Jonson,[37] many lay commentators counteract the levity associated with fatness with stern cautions about the ill effects of habitually overeating. John Evans, for example, collected both witticisms and warnings about the results of eating too much in his commonplace book, which he organized by alphabetized topics. Under "F," he quotes jokes about a fat woman from Shakespeare's Comedy of Errors ("I know not what use to put her to [but] make a lamp of her, & run from her by her own light" and "Spherical like a globe, I would find out whole countries in her").[38] His entry under "S" for surfeiting, however, takes on a far more serious tone. He quotes an author referred to only as HW to caution that many "By surfeiting digged their graves with their own teeth."[39] Given the immense social significance attached to public feasts and banquets in the early modern period, however, the effects of overindulgence were often visible in the bodies of those eager to demonstrate their class status.[40] Jane Huggett suggests that vanity might have provoked some great eaters to take up slimming regimens, citing a poem by Henry Fitz-Geoffrey written in 1617 that makes reference to a young gallant who will:

> ... have an attractive lace
> And whalebone-bodice, for the better grace;
> Admit spare diet; or no substance feed
> But oatmeal, milk and crumbs of barley-bread;
> Use exercise until at last he fit
> (With much ado) his body into it.[41]

Printed medical manuals, too, sometimes contain recipes that reference a patient's body size. *A verye excellent and profitable booke conteining sixe hundred foure score and odde experienced medicines* (1569), a translation of Girolamo Ruscelli's larger work *Secreti nuovi*, offers a recipe entitled "To make a lean person to become fat" that is immediately followed by a matching concoction designed "To make a fat person become lean." The placement suggests that these issues, though seemingly opposite, were seen as disparate manifestations of a common concern with body size. Perhaps surprisingly for modern readers, the recipes for both reducing and gaining weight contain honey as a key ingredient; honey, however, was considered to have drying properties, and it also served as a vehicle for delivering other substances that modify the body's internal, heat-driven processes of digestion.[42] For example, the recipe for helping patients gain weight requires that the "seeds of Orobo" (a variety of wild pea) be mixed with honey, and that the patient ingest the resulting compound daily. The recipe for helping a person become lean, on the other hand, instructs the reader to

> Take four ounces of warm Vinegar, and put therein a quantity of the powder of Pepper, and give it unto the party to drink many mornings fasting, and he will become lean, or else give him to drink every morning of the Wine of sour Pomegranates, two scruples with Oxymel, or water.[43]

Oxymel, as the treatise's own marginal gloss explains, "is a medicine made of honey and water sodden together," and while this may not seem a likely weight-loss treatment at first glance, the drying powers of pomegranate would certainly, in the Renaissance mind, counteract the potential damage that modern readers might see caused by the honey.[44] Pepper and vinegar, meanwhile, increase heat while also helping to dry out the overly moist interior of the overweight body. William Bulleyn even goes so far in his printed health manual as to condemn the habitual use of these last two ingredients, arguing in his printed volume that "artificial women" often "eat pepper, dried corn, and drink vinegar, with such like baggage, to dry up their blood" and to keep their bodies trim.[45]

The Stanhope family receipt book offers a different set of treatments for altering body size, apparently designed to work together, under the heading "To prevent fatness, or to make fat folk lean." These too call on honey and pepper as active ingredients, though they also reflect some of the less complicated approaches the era's recipes held toward weight loss:

1. take six drachmas of sandaracha and drink it in the morning with faire water and oxymel.[46]
2. Also take the rinds of yellow myrobalans, (roast them as though they were burnt) a quarter of an ounce make them to fine powder and drink it in plantain water. [47]
3. Also take a crust of bread, and vinegar and pepper every morning but if you fear it hurt your sinews forbear it.[48]

The third recipe suggests what was also a common Renaissance trick to weight loss, that of eating bread with the idea of drying out the body's interior. William Vaughan writes of this approach's popularity when he notes that "some say" biscuits and crackers "causeth fat people to be lean"; he goes on to endorse the approach himself, noting that these foods "dryeth a moist body, and hinder fatness and all diseases proceeding from moisture, because it keepeth the meat from being too suddenly and quickly conveyed into all the parts of the body."[49] The logic resembles that of today's high-fiber diets, with the full feelings of absorbent bread working in conjunction with a labored digestive process that keeps the body from feeling empty too quickly.

By far the most commonly mentioned approach to weight loss, however, is the most straightforward. Herbs, often in the form of teas, appear to have been the most universally accepted means of achieving bodily leanness, with fennel as the most commonly invoked cure for such purposes. Lady Frances Catchmay offers a selection of recipes "for shortness of Breath, and fatness of the body"; in particular, she suggests fennel tea upon waking in the morning, adding that the patient might sop bread in the mixture as well.[50] Jane Jackson's book prescribes a similar fennel tea for "him that hath a great body and swollen at the stomach."[51] Her second mention of this treatment is more specific regarding the preparation of the tea, directing the reader to "Take the leaves of fennel[,] boil in water that the strength be in it[,] then drain it through cloth and drink of it in the morning fasting and when you go to bed and in wine if you will."[52] While the process of administering the cure is more detailed, the proportions of fennel to water are left for the reader to deduce. The manuscripts may omit the specifics on the assumption that doses would vary to the individual patients' needs, or that the reader would already have a sense of the procedures involved in following the prescription. Such factors, however, do not prevent Jackson from offering more particular directions in later instructions regarding body size. In fact, Jackson prescribes different treatments for men and women when relating her final two recipes. She instructs readers to mix together a concoction of cinnamon, rhubarb, and ginger to relieve the sufferings of "a man that hath a great belly"; to treat a woman in the same shape, readers should "Take polypodium [ferns] that groweth upon an oak as much as will stuff a young pullet and seethe them in two gallons of faire water" along with licorice, and have the patient drink it first thing in the morning and before bed.[53]

Some manuscripts are even more explicit in their considerations of the patient's individual constitution, often insisting that the dose of a given prescription depends upon the patient's body size. A medical manuscript at the Folger Shakespeare Library, for example, describes a water designed to treat those suffering from either plague or surfeit. "[I]t is to be taken blood warm," the recipe instructs, before specifying "for a man" a dose of "12 spoonfuls with sugar." For children, the recipe continues, a "less proportion" should be given "according to the bigness of the p[ar]ty."[54] While the difference between a child and a man contains a great many variables, and though the recipe offers no specifics as to how a woman's treatment should be administered, the direction clearly factors body size into the prescription. The notion of working with "proportion" is particularly interesting, revealing an awareness not just of the importance of scaling down ingredients for patients of particular ages, but for taking into consideration the effects of certain body sizes on a treatment's success.

## WOMEN AS ARBITERS OF APPETITE

In one of the more remarkable instances of household prescriptions concerning body size, it appears that herbs need not actually be ingested to be seen as effective in influencing an individual's eating. The second part of Ruscelli's treatise contains the following tip, under the heading "To make that a woman shall eat of nothing that is set upon the table," for those eager to keep women of the household from overindulging: "Take a little green Basil, and when men bring the dishes to the table, put it under-

neath them, that the woman perceive it not: for men say that she will eat
of none of that which is in the dish where under the Basil lyeth."[55] The
recipe's distinctive quality stems from more than its seeming lack of
underlying scientific justification. Unlike most other medical advice dis-
pensed in the volume, this recipe specifically makes gender a factor, claiming that hidden basil will only be effective in repelling women eaters. As
usual, the book offers no explanation for the cure, nor does it offer any
indication as to why such a cure might be valuable. Instead, it leaves readers to assume that at times it is simply necessary to keep women from
eating particular dishes. Though the question of body size never directly
arises, it is tempting to conclude that the issue would be a factor. What is
most striking is that the cure can be administered to a woman without her
awareness, suggesting that dietary choices can be secretly imposed upon
eaters at a particular table. As a result, readers learn that they can control
a woman's appetite without her knowledge, gaining her unwitting cooper-
ation in a treatment about which she may know nothing, or from which
she may have otherwise rebelled. Placing basil under a plate thus functions as a means of controlling a woman's appetite—and of influencing
her body size—while she remains ignorant of the plan, suggesting that,
when it came to eating habits, women may not have always followed the
advice of those who served food in the household. The recipe thus explicitly gives the women who plan, cook, and serve meals, along with any
male readers who happen upon this printed cure, the power to impose
their will on other women in the arena of food and eating.

Given the existence of such a recipe, it appears that a woman's eating
habits, health, and body size proved significant enough to compel a sneaky
imposition of dieting. The medical reasons for monitoring a woman's body
size were manifold, and they often blended with social expectations of
female behavior. The obese body, after all, was long associated with a wide
variety of uncontrolled appetites. As Gail Kern Paster has shown, a
woman's inability to control her own body subjected her to public humiliation, marking her character as immodest and her flesh permeable, specifically to sexual temptation. She becomes an example of the Bakhtinian
grotesque body, one that cannot control its own urges and functions and
that indulges its fleshly desires regardless of the restrictive social mores that
might surround it.[56] Culturally, a woman's willingness to indulge her
appetite for food suggests a parallel craving for sexual activity, though,
strangely enough, such yearnings need not mark her as fertile. The issue of
body size intertwines with the image of the pregnant woman when it
comes to printed books, and their male authors often make the connection in surprising ways. According to Ruscelli, for example, a woman's
appetite for food could interfere with her fertility, leading to obesity rather

than to pregnancy; his book prescribes an herbal broth of betony to cure "women which through fatness can not conceive."[57] The recipe reflects a conviction that indulgence in food marks a woman as available in culturally inappropriate ways, designating her as a consumer rather than as a fertile producer of future generations.

Printed medical manuals, whose authors were overwhelmingly male in the early modern period, routinely emphasized women's roles as consumers, rather than providers, of both food and of medical care. Pregnancy is one of the few instances in which these publications identify a patient's gender, and in the recorded scenarios female bodies are often imagined as suffering from ravenous, undeniable appetites. Andrew Boorde, for example, states in his book *The Brevarie of Health* that "An unnatural appetite is to eat and drink at all times without due order, or to desire to eat raw and unlawful things, as women with child doth and such like." He offers only a half-hearted remedy for these pregnancy cravings in women, too, saying only, "I have known [that] such lusts hath been put away by smelling to the savour of their own shoes, when they be put off. In such lusts it is best [that] women have their desire if it may be gotten, for they shall never take surfeit by such lusts."[58]

On the home front, though, it was women who determined whether to administer such cures, and they were also the ones who determined whether a particular person's appetite fell outside the realm of expected, acceptable behavior, thus demanding treatment. Home medical manuscripts, for example, acknowledge that pregnant women can indeed suffer from potentially harmful cravings, yet their treatments prove milder and perhaps more useful. Under the heading "To put a woman with child from her Longings," a Folger Shakespeare Library manuscript records the following straightforward cure: "Take a wine glass [full] of spring water [and have her] drink it, and if that will not cure[,] another."[59]

The position that women enjoyed as overseers of both eating and medical care in the household gave them the power to control not just their own bodies—ones that often seem out of control in the printed books—but those of men and other women as well. The household manuscripts that these women often turned to reflect this position of power, addressing readers in a way that respected their ability to exercise control in household matters. While these medical manuscripts were valuable in the daily working of Renaissance households, their contents rarely circulated beyond the neighborhood. The women who wrote them kept their medical practices within their communities, never seeking to publish their medical books for public consumption. As household medical books and their recipes circulated through private channels, women created their own area of food-centered health-care expertise at a time when men were trying to secure their authority over the medical professions. As Hunter shows, the founding of the Society of Apothecaries in 1617 functioned in part as an attempt to remove the arts of distillery and pharmacy from the home and from women's control. As a result, she argues, printed books "begin to show evidence of a distinct split between food as cookery and food as medicine, and between herbal preparations as medicine and chemical preparations as medicine."[60]

But this move also secured female control over cookery, domesticating dietary health practices rather than professionalizing them. In short, this step toward professionalizing medical care granted women more control over food and food-based health-care treatments than ever before. With this control over the kitchen, women retained their influence over the bodies of those in their household. Their practices might have fallen less easily into the era's definition of medicine, but women's oversight of food preparation—and consumption—in their households also granted them power to monitor the diets, health, and resulting body sizes of their family members. Such concerns regarding obesity, lost appetite, and food consumption were not of immediate concern to the university-trained physicians who were increasingly regulating medical practice in cities and in the public realm of print, yet these issues appear to have remained meaningful parts of health care in the home. In their daily practices, then, women oversaw both the production of their households' foods and the health of the bodies that this food helped to nurture.

The household manuscripts these women consulted in turn reveal integral connections among health, eating habits, and patient body size. Blending cookery and health care, home medical manuals reveal that, in matters of everyday practice, body size and physical health could not be so easily separated, and that the women who served as the first line of defense against illness held a keen awareness of the interplay between these supposedly separate matters. Concerns for nutrition and health intertwine in these books, pointing to an appreciation of the practical implications of body size that rarely received direct mention in male-authored medical manuals that appeared in print, even though many of these manuals' authors emphasized the link between eating and the body's internal humoral balance. Instead, the still-evolving medical establishment's anxiety regarding female control over dietary decisions became encapsulated in printed descriptions of women as prone to gastronomical overindulgence. Ironically, the women who provided most health care in the countryside would never have been aware of these perceptions, since scholarly medical books proved to be such small parts of their worlds. The medical manuals that women wrote, kept, and consulted, however, pay little heed to the notion that their own sex proved so susceptible to the temptations of appetite; instead, these household receipt books concentrated on offering practical advice for physical troubles affecting the health of neighbors, friends, and family. As these manuscript manuals show, body size constituted one of these potential troubles, one that women—with their access to the kitchen and knowledge of food's effect upon the body—were uniquely qualified to treat.[61]

## NOTES

1. Alexander Korda's 1933 film *The Private Life of Henry VIII* undoubtedly holds great responsibility for this image, with Charles Laughton portraying the king tearing apart a chicken, belching, and lamenting, "Refinement's a thing of the past!" See Korda, *The Private Life of Henry VIII*, Video Classics, 1985. For this quotation and more information on Laughton's performance, see Greg Walker, *The Private Life of Henry VIII, The British Film Guide* (London: I. B. Tauris, 2003), 4, 18-26. Images of Henry created during his lifetime show the king in various physical states, from slim to rotund, but the emphasis of these depictions often involves communicating finely-honed political messages rather than capturing the king's physical features. See Margaret Aston, *The King's Bedpost* (Cambridge: Cambridge University Press, 1993).

2. See Jasper Ridley, *Henry VIII* (New York: Viking, 1985), 348-49. By 1540, several diplomats had commented on Henry's girth, saying that his "intemperate eating and drinking" had made him unpredictable and irritable; a suit of armor made for the king around this time measured fifty-four inches around the waist (though this, of course, may not exactly correlate with Henry's size, the suit was remarkably larger than those made in his earlier years).

3. See Nancy Siraisi, *Medieval and Early Renaissance Medicine* (Chicago: University of Chicago Press, 1990), 104-6, for a concise history of Galenic theories, particularly those involving the humors. See Michael Schoenfeldt, "Fables of the Belly in Early Modern England," in *The Body in Parts: Fantasies of Corporeality in Early Modern Europe*, eds. David Hillman and Carla Mazzio (New York: Routledge, 1997), 243-61, for a discussion of the implications Galenic theories brought to individuals' views of their own bodies and inner processes of digestion.

4. Ken Albala, *Eating Right in the Renaissance* (Berkeley: University of California Press, 2002), 7, and see 4-7.

5. See Margaret Pelling, *The Common Lot: Sickness, Medical Occupations and the Urban Poor in Early Modern England* (New York: Longman, 1998) for an exhaustive treatment of health care availability and nutrition among the less privileged.

6. The question of women's literacy in the Renaissance is perplexing and has caused much debate in recent years. In his influential study, David Cressy concludes that "Women were almost universally unable to write their own names for most

of the sixteenth and seventeenth centuries"; based on appearances of "marks" instead of signatures in surviving documents, Cressy calculates a 95 percent illiteracy rate among women during the reign of Elizabeth I. See David Cressy, *Literacy and the Social Order: Reading and Writing in Tudor and Stuart England* (Cambridge: Cambridge University Press, 1980), 145, 176. Recent scholars have questioned his findings; for valuable recaps of these arguments, see Heidi Brayman Hackel, *Reading Material in Early Modern England* (Cambridge: Cambridge University Press, 2005), 56-59, and Jean R. Brink, "Literacy and Education," in *A Companion to English Renaissance Literature and Culture*, ed. Michael Hattaway (Oxford: Blackwell, 2000), 97-99.

7. See Wendy Wall, "Familiarity and Pleasure in the English Household Guide, 1500-1700," in *Staging Domesticity: Household Work and English Identity in Early Modern Drama* (Cambridge: Cambridge University Press, 2002),18-58 for a helpful overview of these books.

8. Sara Pennell, "Introduction," in *Women and Medicine: Remedy Books, 1553–1865,* ed. Sara Pennell (Detroit: Primary Source Media, 2004), [2]. Pennell describes the physical appearance of these books in the introduction to the microfilm collection. This collection of manuscripts from the Wellcome Library for the History and Understanding of Medicine has made receipt books, from the Renaissance and beyond, much more available. The books were seldom published in the Renaissance, though as Lynette Hunter notes, the late seventeenth century saw a boom in household books printed for women. See Lynette Hunter, "Women and Domestic Medicine: Lady Experimenters, 1570-1620," in *Women, Science and Medicine 1500–1700: Mothers and Sisters of the Royal Society*, ed. Lynette Hunter and Sarah Hutton (London: Sutton, 1997), 89.

9. Lady Frances Catchmay, *A book of medicens*, c. 1625, 46, ms. 184a, in *Women in Medicine*, ed. Sara Pennell (Detroit: Primary Source Media, 2004) and Jane Jackson, *A very shorte and compendius Method of Phisicke and Chirurgery*, (1642), 34r, ms 373, in *Women in Medicine*, ed. Sara Pennell (Detroit: Primary Source Media, 2004). I have modernized spellings for all direct quotations from early modern sources.

10. Albala, *Eating*, 5, 177. In a subsequent essay that traces weight loss as a growing concern in medical literature after 1650, Albala provides a succinct study of Renaissance approaches to fat. These include a fascinating account of humoral medical explanations regarding the accumulation of fat in the body, as well as cautions regarding sudden shifts in diet. On the whole, though, Albala maintains in the essay that before 1650, "practical dietary writers were still silent on the subject of fat." See Albala, "Weight Loss in the Age of Reason," in *Cultures of the Abdomen: Diet, Digestion, and Fat in the Modern World*, ed. Christopher E. Forth and Ana Carden-Coyne (New York: Palgrave, 2005), 172.

11. Emanuel Van Meteren, "Pictures of the English in Queen Elizabeth's Reign," in *England as Seen by Foreigners in the Days of Elizabeth and James I*, ed. William Brenchley Rye, 1865, reprint (New York: Benjamin Blom, 1967), 72.

12. See Sara Pennell, "Perfecting Practice?: Women, Manuscript Recipes and Knowledge in Early Modern England," in *Early Modern Women's Manuscript Writing: Selected Papers from the Trinity/Trent Colloquium*, ed. Victoria E. Burke and Jonathan Gibson (Aldershot: Ashgate, 2004), 243.

13. Hunter, "Women and Domestic Medicine," 93, 100.

14. Hilary Spurling, *Elinor Fettiplace's Receipt Book: Elizabethan Country Home Cooking* (New York: Viking, 1986), 20, 18. This proportion, along with the seeming lack of recipes for everyday meals, leads C. Anne Wilson to doubt that the book was Fettiplace's chief household guide. Instead, she argues that the book represented Fettiplace's early expertise in confectionary and distillery, two areas to which girls would have been introduced before learning cookery proper from their mothers. See C. Anne Wilson, "A Cookery-Book and Its Context: Elizabeth Cookery and Lady Fettiplace," *Petits propos culinaires* 25 (1987): 8–12.

15. See Margaret Hoby, *Diary of Lady Margaret Hoby: 1599–1605*, ed. Dorothy M. Meads (London: Routledge, 1930), 72, 77, 100.

16. The book's genealogy is recorded in great detail in Spurling, *Elinor Fettiplace's Receipt Book*, 34–37, and abbreviated in Wilson, "A Cookery-Book," 7.

17. Rebecca Price, *The Compleat Cook, or The Secrets of a Seventeenth Century Housewife*, ed. Madeline Masson and Anthony Vaughan, (London: Routledge, 1974), 345, as quoted in Pennell, "Perfecting," 240.

18. Pennell reveals that Nicholas Blundell's diary makes note of several men writing and organizing their wives' recipes. See Pennell, "Introduction," [11]. Also see Pennell, "Perfecting," 241, for a further example. The scribe responsible for copying recipes into Lady Fettiplace's book is known to be Anthony Bridges. See Spurling, *Elinor Fettiplace's Receipt Book*, 21–22. For further information, see Pennell, "Perfecting," 242, as well as the list of manuscript attributions in the contents section of the microfilmed Wellcome collection, where men's names are occasionally used as labels for family manuscripts.

19. For a full discussion of the factors contributing to manuscript compilation, see Pennell, "Introduction," [11–13]. In the case of medicinal recipes, Pennell argues that notes regarding a particular treatment's sources carry the authority of "the 'professional' position of men or the elevated state of women who contributed cures." See Pennell, "Perfecting," 251. Spurling offers a list of doctors whose prescriptions and procedures are recorded in Lady Fettiplace's receipt book; she specifies that William Shakespeare's physician son-in-law proves the source of many treatments. See Spurling, *Elinor Fettiplace's Receipt Book*, 18–19.

20. Fettiplace's book has an added index, for example. See Spurling, *Elinor Fettiplace's Receipt Book*, 21. There are also occasions when she made notes for future users to show modifications she adopted in the recipes. See Wilson, "A Cookery-Book," 16–17. Pennell also notes that books often contain multiple recipes for a particular dish or treatment, and that owners sometimes added

notes cautioning future readers to adjust ingredient amounts or to forego making a particular recipe altogether. See Pennell, "Perfecting," 245, 247-50.

21. Speaking of culinary recipes, Jean-Francois Revel comments that the directions found in early modern household manuals are "far removed from the finished product. Between the two there lies the indefinable domain of tricks and knacks and basic tastes that are always implicit, never explained in so many words, because the books are addressed to people who speak the same language." *Revel, Culture and Cuisine: A Journey through the History of Food* (Garden City: Doubleday, 1982), 12, as quoted in Pennell, "Perfecting," 238.

22. See Katherine Packer, *A book of very good medicines for several diseases wounds and sores both new and olde* (1639), ms. V.a. 387, Folger Shakespeare Library, Washington, DC, 82. In most household medical books, digestive herbs are usually steeped to make teas or tonics; rarely are proportions given.

23. The evolution of recipe forms has earned a great deal of attention from scholars of both household practices and hard sciences. Tebeaux suggests that recipes in seventeenth-century printed cookbooks "became longer and more elaborate, their sentence structures more developed and their recipes more complex than those published in the first half of the sixteenth century." See Elizabeth Tebeaux, "Women and Technical Writing, 1475-1700: Technology, Literacy and Development of a Genre," in *Women, Science and Medicine 1500–1700*, ed. Lynette Hunter and Sarah Hutton (London: Sutton, 1997), 33-35. In his discussion of printed scientific and household manuals, Eamon argues that a recipe is in fact inherently experimental, a "prescription for taking action" that can be tested but is never completely self-contained. See William Eamon, *Science and the Secrets of Nature: Books of Secrets in Medieval and Early Modern Culture* (Princeton: Princeton University Press, 1994), 130-33. Pennell argues that instructions for health-care preparations seem to exhibit precision sooner than cookery recipes, noting that "formal medical prescriptions" often appeared alongside remarkably less structured recipes in household manuscripts. See Pennell, "Introduction," [7], note 7.

24. Philip Stanhope, *A Booke of severall receipts*, (c. 1635), ms. 762, in *Women in Medicine*, ed. Pennell, 203r. Wilson argues that sugar was evidently considered a medicinal rather than a culinary ingredient for much of the Renaissance. See Wilson, "Sugar: The Migrations of a Plant Product during 2000 Years," *Food in Motion, Proceedings of the Oxford Symposium* (Stanningley, Leeds: Prospect Books, 1983), quoted in Wilson, "A Cookery-Book," 13.

25. *A book of receipts which was given me by several men for several causes, griefs, and diseases* . . . (c. 1625-c. 1700), ms. V.a.361-62, Folger Shakespeare Library, 12 v.

26. John Partridge, *Treasuries of commodious conceits*, B3r, London, 1600; see page E1v of the Folger copy for the inscription of ownership.

27. *A book of receipts which was given me by several men for several causes, griefs, and diseases*. . . ., 5r.

28. Packer, *A book of very good medicines*, 15.

29. *A book of receipts which was given me by severall men for severall causes, griefs, and diseases....*, 17v and 6r.

30. Sarah Long, *Mrs. Sarah Longe her Receipt Booke*, c. 1610, ms. V.a.425, Folger Shakespeare Library, Washington, DC, 31r and 41r.

31. See Albala, *Eating*, 55–56. Indeed, Albala notes that the Renaissance concern with lapsed appetite is "hard to assess," speculating that perhaps learned dietary guides paid so much attention to the issue because of the warmer Mediterranean climates in which the books originated or simply as the result of medical fads.

32. Jackson, *A very shorte and compendius Method*, 26v and 87r.

33. *Medical miscellany* (c. 1634), ms. E.a.5, Folger Shakespeare Library, Washington, DC, 58r.

34. Packer, *A book of very good medicines*, 38.

35. Clifford remarks on one occasion, "I kept so ill a Diet with Mrs. Carey & Mrs. Kinson on eating Fruit so that I shortly fell into...sickness" and on another that while visiting a friend she "ate so much cheese there that it made me sick." See Anne Clifford, *The Diaries of Lady Anne Clifford*, ed. D. J. H. Clifford (Phoenix Mill: Sutton, 1990), 26, 57–8.

36. Katherine Paston, *The Correspondence of Lady Katherine Paston, 1603–1327*, ed. Ruth Hughey, vol. 14 (Norfolk: Norfolk Record Society, 1941), 78.

37. See Bruce Thomas Boehrer, *The Fury of Men's Gullets: Ben Jonson and the Digestive Canal* (Philadelphia: University of Pennsylvania Press, 1997) for a fascinating treatment of Ben Jonson and food.

38. John Evans, *Hesperides, or the Muses Garden* (1655–1659), ms. V.b.93, Folger Shakespeare Library, 292. Dromio of Syracuse states these lines regarding his "wondrous fat marriage" at 3.2.95–96 and 113–14 of William Shakespeare, *The Comedy of Errors*, in *The Norton Shakespeare*, ed. Stephen Greenblatt, 2nd ed. (New York: Norton, 2008).

39. Evans, 753.

40. See Stephen Mennell, *All Manners of Food: Eating and Taste in England and France from the Middle Ages to the Present* (Urbana: University of Illinois Press, 1996), and Chris Meads, *Banquets Set Forth: Banqueting in Renaissance Drama* (Manchester: Manchester University Press, 2001) for more on the significance of public celebratory meals.

41. Jane Huggett, *The Mirror of Health: Food, Diet and Medical Theory, 1450–1660* (Bristol: Stuart Press, 1995), finds these lines in her reading of Gerald Eades Bentley, though she offers no citation for the quotation and I have not been able to find her source. Quoted in Huggett, 47–48.

42. See Albala, *Eating*, 86. Albala explains that honey was considered hot and dry, the ideal combination for revving up the digestive process.

43. Girolamo Ruscelli, *A verye excellent and profitable booke conteining sixe hundred foure score and odde experienced medicines, apperteyning unto phisick and surgerie, long tyme practysed of the expert and Reuerend Mayster Alexis, which he termeth the fourth and finall booke of his secretes.... Translated out of Italian into Englishe by Richard Androse* (London, 1569), 38. While there are earlier English language translations, I quote this one because the Folger Shakespeare Library's copy, bound with the first and third parts of Ruscelli's treatise, was owned at one point by a woman.

44. In its definition of oxymel, the OED, "notes that vinegar is usually a required ingredient in the mixture. Vaughan describes the pomegranate as "drying." William Vaughan, *Directions for Health both Naturall and artificiall* (London, 1617), 101.

45. William Bulleyn, *A newe booke entitled the governement of healthe* (London, 1558), C15r, quoted in Albala, *Eating*, 152. Albala also explains that many medical authorities saw vinegar as "lightening" the body through its acidic properties. See *Eating*, 77.

46. While the only uses of the word "sandaracha" in the OED refer to red arsenic sulfide, a chemical used as a pigment and in fireworks, "sandarac" refers to either a tree gum used to create varnish, or, more appetizingly, to honeycomb.

47. The OED explains that a myrobalan is an "astringent plumlike fruit"; it can refer to the fruits of a variety of trees.

48. Stanhope, *A Booke of severall receipts*, 206r.

49. William Vaughan, *Directions for Health*, 33. Albala makes reference to this source in *Eating*, and adds in "Weight Loss" that Tobias Venner advocated a similar use of biscuit. See *Eating*, 95, and "Weight Loss," 172.

50. Catchmay, *A book of medicens*, 62v.

51. Jackson, *A very shorte and compendius Method*, 35r.

52. Ibid., 36r.

53. Ibid., 119v.

54. *Medical Recipes* (1600–1610), ms. E.b.1, Folger Shakespeare Library, 1v.

55. Ruscelli, *The seconde parte of the Secrets of maister Alexis of Piemont* (London, 1568), 14r. This book is bound with other books of Ruscelli's treatise in the Folger Shakespeare Library's copy.

56. See Gail Kern Paster, *The Body Embarrassed* (Ithaca: Cornell University Press, 1993), 1–22.

57. Ruscelli, *A verye excellent and profitable book*, 36v.

58. Andrew Boorde, *The Breuiary of helthe* (London, 1547), xix r to xix v. Boorde's book underwent several reprintings in the Renaissance, the latest in 1598.

59. *A book of receipts which was given me by severall men*, 29r.

60. Hunter, "Women and Domestic Medicine," 96.

61. I wish to thank the Faculty Research Committee of The University of Akron for the financial support that made this research possible, as well the Friends of the University Libraries at The University of Akron for their willingness to purchase materials for this project. Jason M. Demeter and K. E. Birdsall also offered much appreciated help in preparing this chapter for publication.

TWO

# Remapping Maternity in the Courtroom

## *Female Defenses and Medical Witnesses in Eighteenth-Century Infanticide Proceedings*

SHEENA SOMMERS

DURING THE EIGHTEENTH CENTURY, ENGLISH courts began to acquit women accused of newborn infant murder in numbers not previously seen.[1] Whereas seventeenth-century women accused of infanticide were generally portrayed within the courtroom as "monstrous mothers" *par excellence*, eighteenth-century trial records rely heavily upon new narratives that represent the accused as a helpless victim of circumstance. Female defenses for infanticide during this period became increasingly elaborate renditions of their sufferings, and courts inquired ever more into the emotional state of the accused. By the second half of the eighteenth century, internal states of mind such as being out of one's senses at the time of delivery replaced other forms of defenses for infanticide that had been based more firmly upon material evidence such as the preparation of linen by the accused.[2]

As surgeons and male midwives began to replace female midwives as the key trial witnesses, the "truth" of these cases was increasingly sought through the dissections performed on the infant's corpse. Despite the fundamental inconclusiveness of medical testing, the findings from dissections were, more often than not, used by the courts to validate the new defenses of nonresponsibility. Thus, medical evidence became crucial to these trials for reasons other than its ability to offer reliable scientific determinations.

The child's body came to function in these cases as the privileged site through which the suffering of the accused could be uncovered and explained, using the authority of medical discourse to legitimate highly sympathetic accounts of the mother's travails, which worked to exonerate her from guilt.

The role of expert testimony in court proceedings was not new to the eighteenth century. Dating back to the fourteenth century, individuals possessing expertise were called upon to act as special advisors to the court.[3] During the seventeenth century, however, expert witnesses began to be called not as adjudicators, or private advisors to the court, but rather as witnesses whose testimony was to be evaluated, like that of other witnesses, by a lay jury.[4] Changes in legal practice during the eighteenth century, including an increasingly adversarial system, a growing demand for certainty and standards of proof to obtain conviction, and a heightened focus upon circumstantial evidence, all contributed to the rise of expert witness testimony.[5] According to Stephen Landsman, the growing need for certainty within the judicial process contributed to a general devaluation of direct (lay) testimony in favor of the circumstantial evidence offered by "disinterested medical witnesses."[6] In infanticide trials in particular, the problems of ascertaining proof in cases of secret births made the role of expert witnesses particularly crucial as circumstantial evidence was generally all that could be obtained in such cases. As almost every woman tried had concealed her pregnancy and given birth alone, medical testing was one of the only means available to the courts with which to make determinations about the state of the child at the time of its birth.

Medical experts were most frequently brought in by the courts rather than by the defense or prosecution and had generally already been involved in the case through the dissection of the body in the case of surgeons, or through the examination of the mother's body in the case of midwives. As such, their testimony was, in theory, that of an informed yet impartial witness. Obvious partisanship was condemned by the courts despite the fact that judges frequently exerted pressure upon medical witnesses to provide conclusive statements.[7] The increasingly adversarial nature of the eighteenth-century legal process altered the judge's role in the trial. By the latter part of the century, rather than engaging as inquisitors themselves, judges more often took on the role of clarifying the findings of medical experts and testing their conclusions.[8] The witness' description of experiments made upon the corpse, although usually uncertain, nevertheless allowed the medical experts to present their findings as objective facts while simultaneously allowing the courts flexibility in their interpretation of the validity of such experiments. The general increase in reliance upon experimental proof during the eighteenth century at once validated the authority of professional medical witnesses while at the same time devaluating traditional forms of testimony offered by both lay witnesses and female midwives.

The more rigorous standards of proof as well as the flexibility with which medical evidence could be interpreted by judges and juries enabled eighteenth-century courts to acquit women accused of infanticide despite the legal intent of the 1624 Statute. In the highly ambiguous arena of secret births, definitive truths about the body—about what was possible and what was not—were almost impossible to come by. It was precisely the inherent uncertainty surrounding these cases, the secrecy and privacy of the crime itself, that had helped to justify the implementation of a particularly draconian statute against infanticide. The English Act to Prevent the Destroying and Murdering of Bastard Children stated specifically that any unmarried woman

> Be[ing] delivered of any issue of her body, male or female, which being born alive, should by the laws of this realm be a bastard, and that she endeavour privately, either by drowning or secret burying thereof, or any other way, either by herself or the procuring of others, so to conceal the death thereof, as that it may not come to light, such case the said mother so offending shall suffer death as in the case of murther, except such mother can make proof by one witness at the least, that the child (whose death was by her so intended to be concealed) was born dead.[9]

The severity of the legal statute effectively placed the burden of proof upon the defendant as it made "concealment of the delivery of an illegitimate child" who was later found dead proof positive of infanticide unless there was one witness who could proclaim that the infant had not in fact been born alive.[10] The wording of the statute worked to counter some of the evidentiary difficulties involved in ascertaining proof of murder in cases of secret births as women were charged for concealment of pregnancy rather than for murder.[11]

There is ample evidence to suggest that eighteenth-century English courts, unlike their seventeenth-century predecessors, were increasingly unwilling to prosecute and convict women accused of newborn infant murder.[12] Recent scholarship reveals that this trend was occurring across Western Europe, with infanticide convictions declining sharply during this period.[13] A romanticization of motherhood and motherly love, a general increase in humanitarian sentiment, as well as a feeling among judges, juries, and legal reformers that the statute governing newborn infant murder was too draconian, have all been put forth by historians as explanations for this decline. J. M. Beatti argues, for instance, that the most significant factor in the decline in convictions for this crime was the "change in attitudes towards the unmarried mother" as indicated by the advent of charitable institutions such as the lying-in hospitals.[14] Peter Hoffer and N. E. C. Hull have suggested that the law itself was increasingly viewed as anachronistic and out of step with a culture more interested in the sentimental aspects of mothering.[15]

Nevertheless, according to Mark Jackson, most scholarship to date has relied upon a vaguely defined "reform perspective," where it is assumed that a general increase in humanitarian feeling inspired lighter sentencing by the courts.[16] While Jackson does not wholly deny this as one of the possibilities for the decreasing rate of convictions, he calls for greater attention to be paid to the role of medical discourse and the increasing tendency of courts to focus on detailed, scientific, "natural explanations" as a way to understand these seemingly "unnatural crimes."[17]

Thomas Laqueur likewise suggests that the eighteenth century saw the birth of a new narrative habit that linked detailed, objective knowledge as a sign of truth (including the body as a site of scientific discourse) with the "suffering subject," to produce what he terms the "humanitarian narrative."[18] While there are a variety of factors involved in the declining rates of prosecution, relatively little attention has been paid to these "scientific shifts," specifically, the general appropriation of female reproductive knowledge by the medical and scientific community and the subsequent trend toward viewing birth as an essentially passive (in)activity that—particularly in cases of secret births—could only be made sense of by recourse to the objective professionalism of male medical learning. As experiential knowledge became increasingly suspect, male medical practitioners were positioned by the courts—and positioned themselves—as the necessary interpreters of the body. The language of scientific objectivity lent these witnesses an aura of authority despite the fact that their testimony was frequently speculative and their evidence uncertain.[19]

While male witnesses and surgeons drew heavily upon women's own stories of secret births and were quite frequently willing to utilize their evidence to create and validate highly sympathetic accounts on behalf of the accused, their very existence within the courtroom worked to challenge the traditional female domain of experiential knowledge and authority. As medical evidence was increasingly used by judges and surgeons to legitimate female defenses of senselessness and vulnerability, the testimony of these men served as a reminder of their importance not only in courtrooms but also in lying-in chambers. The absence of these men in the former might result in judicial confusion, yet their absence in the latter—as documented by the tragic events of these proceedings—had far more severe consequences, namely the inevitability of infant death in cases of unattended births.

## WOMEN'S DEFENSES IN THE COURTROOM

Female narratives concerning secret births were malleable creations and women's confessions shifted throughout the process of investigation and exposure. Accused women drew upon a number of defenses including, but not limited to: marriage; the defense of linen; early onset deliveries; senselessness during labor; and falls and frights before the birth that led to stillborn infants. As the eighteenth century wore on, successful defenses combined a large number of these claims, weaving them into recognizable forms designed to provoke sympathy from judges and juries. Narrative strategies became much more detailed and complex during this period and, as Dana Rabin argues, increasingly referred to the "emotional or mental state of the accused" as a "primary explanation for the crime."[20]

The most common line of defense used at the Old Bailey Courthouse at the beginning of the eighteenth century was the defense of linen. From 1700 to 1725, the preparation of linen was used as evidence in favor of the accused in approximately 55 percent of defenses. Only one of the women who proved she had prepared for the birth in this way was found guilty under the statute. While only a small number of guilty verdicts were returned overall, linen was an important component of the court's decision to acquit. Women like Ann Hasle, tried in 1717, who could produce a "considerable quantity of child-bed linen" in court stood a greater chance of acquittal than those women who could not.[21] Thus, in Ann Morris's trial at the Old Bailey in 1722, the midwife deposed that when she asked the accused if she had provided anything for the child, Ann apparently replied, "No indeed, Mrs. Cooper, I've provided nothing." Although Ann's case was quite typical, having disposed of the infant into the "House of Ease," without any outward signs of harm upon the child's body, the midwife's evidence was taken seriously by the courts and Ann was subsequently sentenced to death.[22] Likewise, Ann Gardner, tried in 1708, had little to say in her defense, and as it "did not appear that she made any Provision for the Birth of a Child" the statute was read out in court, and she was found guilty of the indictment.[23]

Linen continued to be an important component of defenses during the second quarter of the century as well. From 1726 to 1750, the use of linen as a defense had dropped slightly, to just over 45 percent, although courts continued to inquire into this fact and utilize this as evidence in their determination of guilt. The second most often used defense during the first half of the eighteenth century was claiming to have come before one's time. During the first quarter of the century this was used in 35 percent of defense narratives and by the second quarter in 30 percent of the cases. Mary Gough, tried in 1719, told the court that she "reckoned she had 6 Weeks longer to go." While both the midwife and surgeon in her case believed upon examination that the child was born at full term, Gough was acquitted of the charge.[24] For the judges and juries, whether or not the child had actually been early does not seem to have been the most important consideration. Early delivery defenses suggested rather that the accused had gone into labor unexpectedly, was surprised by the onset of her pains, and was therefore unprepared for the birth of the child. As such, this kind of defense worked to construe labor as a quick, unanticipated event that the accused could neither predict nor control. These defense narratives stressed the woman's helplessness and highlighted the fact that under such dire circumstances there could exist no premeditation for murder.

The combination of the preparation of linen and the early delivery defense worked well within the trial context because it provided the courts with evidence of maternal devotion and suggested a lack of premeditation. Women such as Elizabeth Warner, tried in 1760, seemed to have recognized that such quick and painless labors could be grounds for acquittal. Warner had delivered over the vault (toilet) and while at first telling other witnesses that she had only had a bloody nose, eventually confessed to some neighborhood women that she had in fact been delivered. Elizabeth told the witness, Mary Lawson, that she had come before her time and that the child had "drop'd from her" over the vault with "very little pain." Elizabeth also told a fellow lodger, Margaret Watson, that when she went to the necessary house, in "straining my child came from me." Margaret seemed frightened for Warner, saying, "Lord, Betty, what will you do for the child, for you will be hanged." According to Margaret's testimony, Elizabeth replied, "hanged for what [for] she was come before her time." After numerous failed attempts to get the child out of the vault, Margaret went back upstairs to reproach Warner again, demanding to know how she could do such a thing. Warner begged Margaret not to "reflect" too much and again maintained that she "could not help it, she felt no pain." Watson deposed in court that linen had been found and that another woman had agreed to lend Warner a blanket for the child. Warner was found not guilty of the charge with a telling note at the end of the record specifying that she was acquitted "as delivered by surprise."[25]

The combination of these two defenses continued to be an important component of a successful plea throughout the second half of the eighteenth century, although to a lessening extent. From 1751 to 1775, for instance, the prevalence of linen as a defense had dropped slightly, found in only 36 percent of trial defenses. During the last quarter of the century it was explicitly present in only 20 percent of courtroom narratives. Early delivery defenses dropped from a high of 35 percent during the first quarter of the eighteenth century to only 13 percent from 1751 to 1775 and to just over 6 percent of trial defenses from 1776 to 1800. New defenses stressing a woman's inability to save or care for her infant at the time of the delivery became increasingly common. While the early onset of labor highlighted a lack of premeditation, droppings into the vault and sudden fits of senselessness during delivery began to replace this form of defense. Although dropping generally entailed aspects of the early delivery defense— being surprised by labor as in Elizabeth Warner's case above—this particular defense plea went even further in construing the women accused as entirely unable to stop her child from falling from her body. As such, even bruises and other evidence of harm could be interpreted by the courts to be merely the result of falls into the vault or onto a hard floor rather than as an indication of intentional violence.

While "droppings" were present in less than 5 percent of cases from 1674 to 1700, such a defense increased steadily over the course of the eighteenth century, to 10 percent of cases during the first quarter of the century, then to 27 percent from 1726 to 1750 and to 30 percent during the third quarter.[26] From 1776 to 1800, dropping was the most commonly used component of a defense, present in 33 percent of all trials. Similarly, senselessness during the time of labor, present in none of the late seventeenth-century trials, rose to 8 percent during the first quarter of the century, staying roughly the same at 7 percent from 1726 to 1750, and then rose again to 20 percent of defenses for the rest of the century. Such drastic increases in the prevalence of droppings and senselessness as defense strategies suggest that there were some fairly significant changes in the way in which the process of birth and delivery was described by women and interpreted by the courts. The courts increased allowance for defenses that, strictly speaking, should not have gained women an acquittal when tried under the statute, and effectively rendered the law, in practice, obsolete. The process of birth was being redefined within the courtroom walls and naturalized as essentially an inactivity that surprised and rendered senseless the women accused. As such, rather than being found guilty for what she had done, the trial records suggest that courts increasingly felt that it was unfair to hold women responsible merely for what they had failed to do under such dire circumstances.

The inability of a woman to save her child as it dropped from her body was deemed particularly plausible by the courts when she claimed to have been senseless at the time of her delivery. In Ann Haywood's 1762 trial, she claimed in her defense that when she was "upon the vault a pain came upon me and I could not get off, nor I did not know where I was till I was in bed. I was quite insensible when the child came from me."[27] In 1794, Diana Parker, having apparently admitted to several people that she had put her child down the privy, that "it was born alive" and that she there-fore wished to be brought to justice, developed a different strategy once brought to trial. In court, Diana defended herself by saying that she "did not mean to make away with the child" and that she "did not know what I was about." Diana showed some things that she had made for the child and was subsequently acquitted by the jury.[28] Evidence of cuts, lacerations and bruises upon the child's body could, moreover, be forgiven by the judge and jury if a woman could convince them that she had been out of her mind during her labor. Thus in the cook Sarah Hunter's 1769 trial, her mistress deposed that another servant came to her to tell her that Sarah was "very busy under the bed-clothes" and that she was "doing something to herself" and seemed to have "taken her knife out." The child was discovered the following morning and according to the mistress had a "cut down from the ear, and then another cut across the throat" that seemed to be to right to the "bone of the neck." The surgeon, Mr. Able, likewise described the cut and suggested that the child had been born alive. Despite the severity of the wounds upon the infant's body, Hunter was let off, saying only in her own defense that "I awaked in the morning and found there was a child; that frightened me very much. I was not sensible what I did. I can give no account how I did it."[29]

While it is certainly possible that such defenses were merely conve-nient fictions used by the courts in order to secure acquittal—there is with-out doubt a fairly noticeable lack of concern for the victim of the crime in these cases—they were, nevertheless, most often confirmed by both medical and lay witnesses and, as such, had to fall within the realm of possibility in order to be used by judges and juries in this way. In a culture increasingly interested in notions of sensibility, the moral value of aggrandized feeling, and, particularly, women's more impressionable nature, a woman's sense-lessness could be interpreted as an inherently natural reaction to the calamitous and agonizing circumstances of an unattended birth.[30] These symptoms were increasingly being naturalized, both inside and outside the courtroom, as representative of women's delicate constitution, rather than as indications of mental or physical disease. Whereas insanity pleas in most murder cases were rarely accepted in eighteenth-century legal prac-tice, women's claims to senselessness during delivery were.[31] When medical experts testified to an individual's mental instability in regular cases of murder, the courts, rather than using medical uncertainty to the advantage of the accused, more often utilized the medical witness' inability to provide conclusive statements in order to dismiss the defendant's pleas.[32] Hence, in eighteenth-century criminal proceedings the courts operated within a gendered framework in which the gender of the accused had a fairly signif-icant impact on the court's acceptance of senselessness pleas. The broader cultural discourses surrounding women's more sensitive biological makeup lent a certain plausibility to these defenses within the courtroom.

Thus, even with such a great deal of evidence against women like Hunter, courts continued to return not-guilty verdicts apparently on the grounds of incapacity during the time of delivery. Dropping by itself, without the added component of senseless, could also gain the accused acquittal despite evidence of harm. In Ann Taylor's 1778 trial, the infant's body was examined by a surgeon who found that several of the ribs were cut through and that the head was almost torn off. Mr. Midford, the surgeon, thought that these wounds appeared to have been inflicted with the use of a sharp instrument. The court, however, continued to press Mr. Midford, demanding to know whether or not such wounds could have possibly been the result of the child's dropping into the vault, suggesting to this witness perhaps that the child's body had struck against "the edge of bricks which sometimes project." Mr. Midford was reluctant at first to admit such a possibility, but the court continued to press him until he relented. Midford seems to have been fairly skeptical of the judge's suggestion, but after a lengthy period of questioning the surgeon finally admitted that he "would not say it could not be done so," and in fact he now "believed it might." Mr. Midford's original suspicion that the wounds upon the body of the child were most likely the result of a "cutting instrument" were effectively dismissed by the court on the grounds that Midford could not with certainty discount other possibilities. Ann did not even speak in her own defense, allowing the 'facts' of the case to stand on their own.[33]

The notion that women were much more vulnerable to fits of senselessness has been documented by Roy Porter, who suggests that it was increasingly common to construe women in such a way in advice literature, novels, and medical tracts. He nevertheless argues that such constructions are "remarkable by their absence from letters and journals of men and women faced with the actual circumstances of sickness."[34] Thus, according to Porter, the "age of sensibility produced a great crop of hysterical women, but only between the covers of novels."[35] What is striking, however, is women's own use of these forms of depictions to defend themselves within the courtroom. In the trial context, women were quite willing to draw upon patronizing medical understandings in order to secure their own acquittal. Thus, within eighteenth-century infanticide trials, the fictive representation of the hysterical woman became something of a reality.

## FROM EXPERIENTIAL KNOWLEDGE TO "OBJECTIVITY"

Paralleling the decrease in the incidence of producing linen in court and the rise of defenses of senselessness was the court's increasing reliance on male medical witnesses to decipher the facts of the case. Experiments made by medical witnesses upon the infant's body, while generally inconclusive, were becoming ever more important to judicial inquiries. Throughout the eighteenth century, the child's corpse had been a fairly central piece of evidence; however, in earlier cases from which male practitioners were largely absent, female midwives could only make statements based upon traditional signs of a full-term birth and external evidence of assault or violence found on the body of the child. The growing reliance upon the dissection of the corpse by surgeons in the second half of the century, and the medical testing and terminology that accompanied it, signified a new emphasis upon the body as a source of knowledge.[36] As Jackson maintains, despite popular antagonism toward dissection, the "inspection and dissection of bodies became an increasingly important tool in penetrating the secrets of nature."[37] The escalating scrutiny of evidence found within the infant's corpse can be understood therefore as part of the "novel interest in probing the depths of the human body."[38] While coroner's inquests into suspicious deaths had begun as early as the twelfth century in England, the changes in standards of proof and the greater reliance upon circumstantial evidence during the eighteenth century increased the court's dependence upon scientific experiments, particularly in cases where direct evidence might be difficult or impossible to obtain.[39] Landsman's analysis of eighteenth-century poisoning, rape, and infanticide trials at the Old Bailey—crimes notoriously difficult to prove—reveals that after 1760 the reliance upon lay opinion in court dwindled while recourse to medical expertise rose.[40]

In the case of infanticide the inspection of the mother's body had traditionally provided some insight into the case—for instance, whether or not she had in fact given birth—but as the century progressed the body most closely probed by medical witnesses became that of the infant. It was precisely the findings derived from experiments made upon the corpse that somehow allowed for the creation of narratives that highlighted the experience and suffering of the accused. Thus, although medical evidence centered on the clues found upon or within the corpse, this evidence was used by medical witnesses, often with the consent and even insistence of the courts, to construct hypothetical sequences of illegitimate births that exonerated the accused from responsibility for the death of her infant. The sympathy for the victim of the crime, the child, was therefore transferred to compassion for the suffering of the mother.[41] The child's body became the object of medical testing and the site through which the internal mental and emotional state of the accused at the time of delivery could be ascertained.

While the sharp decline in conviction for infanticide occurred around 1715, male medical witnesses did not become the experts of choice until approximately mid-century. Female midwives were therefore often called upon in these earlier trials to make statements regarding the child's body.

Due to the nature of their practice, however—being barred from the use of instruments, for instance—female midwives could comment only upon the external signs found upon the infant's corpse. Their evidence therefore drew upon traditional tell-tale signs of live or still-births. If the child's fists were open as opposed to clenched, for example, this suggested that the child had been born alive. Thus in 1718, a midwife testified that Ann Mabe's infant was most likely stillborn, for its fists were clenched, and it was her opinion that a "Child that is born new, if alive, came into the World with its Hands expanded; but if dead, with its Hands clench'd."[42] Further evidence included whether or not the infant's fingernails and toe-nails were fully formed, an observation which could be indicative of whether or not a child had been born at full term. The midwife in Deborah Greening's 1725 trial testified therefore that "to the best of her Judgement, the Prisoner did not go her full time, for the Toe Nails of the Infant were not perfect."[43] While such evidence was based upon the signs offered up by the child's body, female midwives, even when sympathetic, rarely went so far as did male practitioners in constructing lengthy and speculative narratives about the events of a secret birth.

While the evidence offered by male witnesses was by no means any more conclusive than that given by female midwives, the use of scientific and medical discourse lent them an aura of authority and helped to lessen at least the semblance of uncertainty that plagued these trials. Thus, while the shift toward the use of male surgeons and midwives cannot be said to have caused the decline in convictions, nor did their medical evidence in effect clarify the "truths" of the case, their increasing presence in these trials suggests that the courts felt that their testimony was somehow vital to the outcome of these trials. While female midwives could certainly utilize the outward signs of the child's body to make statements regarding evidence of full-term births or violence upon the corpse, these external signs did not allow them access to the internal states of mind of the accused, which the male practitioners often assumed. There seems to have been something peculiar to the surgeon's abilities to examine the innards of the body that gave them the propensity to intuit not only a chain of past events from which they were necessarily absent, but also the motivations and feelings of the accused that accompanied her travails. By accessing the innards of the body of the infant, the male practitioner claimed the ability to decipher the internal workings of the mother's mind.

In order to outline the divergent ways in which the body of the dead infant was spoken of and the conclusions that could be drawn from it by male and female practitioners, I will examine two similar cases. In Ann Hullock's 1760 trial, the child was found in the vault with serious injuries. Susannah Dorwood, midwife, described her examination of the child's body in personal and colloquial terms. After taking the child out of the vault the "blood appear'd: I said here is murder committed, the head is almost off; I laid it down on the boards, and it bled prodigiously." The body had been "stuck in the soil, and the soil kept the place [head and body] together, so that the blood had no vent." Dorwood's examination lacks a specific description of the injury as well as a detailed account of how the child may have come by it, except to say here is a murder. Dorwood then confronted the accused and asked her, "How could you lay violent hands on it to draw innocent blood? Do you consider your soul?"[44] Such a direct confrontation between a male practitioner and the accused would have been exceedingly rare. While men were certainly able to draw conclusions about secret births and make judgments surrounding the facts of the case, they rarely "taxed" the accused themselves, leaving this role to women within the community.[45]

In court, however, medical witnesses utilized their examination of the infant's body to assess the facts of the case. In Mary Samuels's 1762 trial, the male midwife George White gives his testimony in a language quite different from Mrs. Dorwood's. Mr. White describes to the court the nature of the injury found upon the infant's body; he explains that it was a "laceration, a tearing by force on the right side of the mouth, beginning at the mouth and extending almost to the ear." Having given the specifics of the injury, unprovoked, he attempts to explain how this might happen, naturally going on to describe how the "poor creature, I doubt not" was in a "great deal of distress, when the child's head might be born, and to extricate herself in that misery, she might introduce her fingers into the child's mouth, she might make use of this means to pull the child from her, which might break the jaw and tear the part." The rationale for his conclusions, while still couched in medical terminology, was nevertheless speculative and sympathetic, as evidenced by his repeated use of the words "she might." Indeed, it is plain to Mr. White that "no person would give themselves pain, if they could help or ease it; every body will try to ease themselves; and as the navel-string was broke before, death [m]ust ensue before the child could be delivered." Although the lungs when immersed in water had floated, suggesting that the child had in fact taken a breath, Mr. White explained to the court that "another of the faculty" agreed with him that even when the "lungs being inflated, and swimming" may suggest a live birth, this is not "always proof of a child's being born alive; that I have had a proof of within these ten days."[46]

While the profusion of blood in the first case may suggest that a narrative such as Mr. White's could not be used, many other cases reveal that even such injuries could be effectively explained away by a sympathetic medical witness. Thus, many infants appeared to have bled to death because the woman was herself unable to tie the umbilical cord properly.[47] The surgeon William Withers confirms this in Sarah Hopkins's trial of 1767, observing that since the navel-string was broken quite close to the navel, he believed from this that the child "could not have lived past a minute or two, but must bleed to death," an event that "might happen as she stood erect."[48] Richard Ingram, a male midwife testifying in Elizabeth Gwatkin's case of 1779, likewise swore that the death of a child "might very easily be accounted for from the umbilical cord not being secured."[49] Again these surgeons are willing to utilize such speculative evidence to suggest that the child died through no fault of the mothers and instead that their ill fates were a result of the mothers' inaction rather than willful action. While female midwives certainly could give testimony suggesting a particularly violent birth, they rarely went beyond these conclusions to reconstruct an entire series of events.[50]

As illustrated by Mr. White's testimony above with regards to the lung test, surgeons were, furthermore, quite willing to discount medical evidence in favor of a narrative of sympathy and suffering. Such a denial of the efficacy of medical testing by surgeons and courts is not uncommon in these trials. The lung test, which involved the removal of the lungs from the infant's body and placing them in water to see if they would float—thus determining whether or not the infant had taken a breath—although fundamental to a surgeon's testimony, was often discounted by either the surgeon himself or by the court. Thus, Robert Young reported in 1762 that after opening the thorax, he took out the lungs

> in order to make the experiment usually made in these cases...the lungs did swim, but I was of the opinion that the experiment cannot be conclusive in this case, because the body had laid 3 days in the bog house, and I think such a fermentation might have been brought off, that it might gather air.[51]

The inconclusiveness of the lung test, although designed to bring greater clarity to these difficult situations, effectively placed the burden of proof upon the prosecution.

In Sarah Russell's trial of 1781, the judge himself tells the surgeon witness that he "understood that the experiment upon the lungs has of late been held not to be conclusive," and that it is only "held to be conclusive, if the lungs sink." The surgeon was obviously compelled to agree with the judge and offered nothing more on the matter except an affirmative "yes."[52] One further example of the court ruling out this evidence is found in the trial of Ann Taylor in 1778. After the jury asked the surgeon Mr. Midford if he dissected the body and performed the usual test, the judge quickly intervened, responding before Mr. Midford had a chance to answer with the claim that, "that is nothing. We never suffer that to be given in evidence."[53]

Findings such as these complicate any simple understanding of the courts' reliance on medical testing as a means to establish the guilt or innocence of the accused. If surgeons and courts themselves increasingly refused to uphold the validity of medical testing, one must ask what purpose such testimony in fact served. The lung test was basically the only evidence that separated the findings of male practitioners from that offered by female midwives. Dissections rarely offered any other substantial evidence as to whether a child had been born alive. By calling into question this test, or by stating, as did the judge in Sarah Russell's case, that it was only held to be conclusive if the lungs sank and therefore substantiated a plea of innocence, the courts in effect made null and void the whole purpose of the surgeon's presence in court. Or did they?

As Laqueur maintains, the "humanitarian narrative" derived its success from its ability to construct "causal chains" of events that connected the "actions of its readers [in this case the judge and jury] with the suffering of its subjects."[54] The dissections of the corpses worked to provide the courts with this necessary connection, making imaginative leaps from the body's signs to the mother's innocence. What surgeons and male medical practitioners offered in these cases was a connection between the innards of the body and the interiority of the feminine mind, accessed by their ability for objective distance, the third term in the mother-child dyad, and related in court within the discourse of medical science. These men's ability to penetrate the truths of the body in ways in which female practitioners could not gave them the authority to draw conclusions about the state of mind of the accused and the sequence of events that she had endured. The child's body became merely a clue to the mother's suffering, and the resulting narrative accounts offered by these medical witnesses, although absolving her from responsibility, increasingly replaced her own voice in the proceedings. Within the courtroom male practitioners were asserting "epistemological sovereignty" over both the "minds and bodies of others."[55] The medical gaze of the distant observer replaced knowledge based upon shared experience, at once objectifying the corpse and simultaneously claiming authoritative entitlement to speak on behalf of the accused.

As the century wore on, sympathetic medical testimony became increasingly common, and midwives either disappeared from the trials or were positioned alongside male medical witnesses in court. Female experiential knowledge was no longer deemed reliable in itself. Indeed, in Elisabeth Gwatkin's 1779 trial, female testimony is directly contradicted and then disregarded by the court in favor of that of the male witnesses. Gwatkin utilized the dropping defense, saying she had been surprised with labor pains while sitting on the vault and that the child fell in. Mr. Jackson, a practitioner of midwifery, when questioned by the court, supported the possibility of such deliveries, testifying that there were "many instances" of such labors. The court asked Mr. Jackson specifically if he thought it possible that a "woman, being at a necessary, upon a needful occasion, may be taken in labour, and for the child to drop from her into the necessary without her putting it there?" Jackson answered that while "I have never known an instance of it; I have frequently heard of its being so." Indeed, he had been previously informed by a lady that her own child had dropped into the necessary and thus Mr. Jackson thought such incidences "very probable."

Contrarily, the witness Elisabeth Bailey, a neighbor of the accused, maintained that she did not believe such births were possible. The court pressed her, suggesting that she herself had said there was a "difference between women." Nevertheless, Bailey retained her original statement. Under cross-examination, however, her testimony was called into question, for, as she had not practiced as a midwife, it followed that "the ground of your [her] observation must be very confined indeed." Bailey replied that she was a married woman herself with children of her own. This fact was, however, no longer enough to persuade the court, for "the possibility of information" that Bailey could have gathered, according to the court, "must be but little." In response to this suggestion Bailey replied that she only answered "according to my judgment." After a third male practitioner was called in and asked again about the possibility of such births, he likewise upheld that he was "clear it [these kind of deliveries] can happen."[56]

While Bailey was not a midwife or medical professional, her answers suggest that she did not feel this fact barred her from making a statement about the case. She was a mother and her experience therefore qualified her to give an opinion. As a married woman, moreover, within the community she most likely maintained the right to express her opinion and exercise a degree of authority in such matters. She was a respectable woman with children who was likely involved in the taxing and searching of the accused, an integral part of the very events that brought Gwatkin to trial. In court, however, Bailey's testimony was easily dismissed by the male medical professionals who, while having no personal experience of birth, were apparently more qualified than she to understand the process of labor. Of course, what is interesting about this case is that while these male medical witnesses would most likely never have seen such a birth—as it generally only happened in the context of concealment of pregnancy and secret deliveries—their evidence draws on (speculative) female experience. Thus, while contradicting the testimony of Elisabeth Bailey, Mr. Jackson nonetheless upholds the validity of such births based upon hearsay, the knowledge reported to him by an anonymous lady.[57] Likewise, all of these male witnesses are in fact legitimating the defenses used by the accused through these medical narratives. Thus, while Bailey's experience as a mother is discounted, Gwatkin's is, ironically, authenticated.

The professional learning of male medical practitioners, by this time, came to outweigh the experiential knowledge of female witnesses even while these men's testimony generally corroborated the defensive strategies of the accused. Not only was Gwatkin acquitted by the courts with the help of these men's testimony, but something else was being created here within the courtroom walls. A new understanding of labor and birth, which rendered certain women incapable of saving their infants from falling out of their bodies and into outhouses, became, throughout the course of the century, increasingly legitimated through legal practice. The tensions between (female) experiential knowledge and (male) objective knowledge were likewise paralleled by the increasingly evident opposition between communal opinion and medical/judicial authority.

While women continued to operate as regulators of sexual morality within the community, their authority in this role was gradually being superseded within the trial setting. By the time of Elizabeth Fletcher's 1747 trial, for instance, the bill was returned *ignoramus*, meaning that, according to the court, there was no case to answer to. The record states tellingly that upon examination of the case, the suspicions directed against Elizabeth appeared to be "entirely without a Foundation, and arose from some poor, ignorant, and rash People, by whose Means this poor Creature was like to fall a Sacrifice to the Mob."[58] While the validity of the neighborhood suspicions could justifiably be brought into question in this case, the tone taken by the jury with regard to the "ignorant mob" is nevertheless significant. Judges and juries, by the second half of the century, not only inquired ever more into the emotional state of the accused at the time of delivery, but moreover positioned themselves as the enlightened protectors of helpless women who were seen as falling victims to the fanaticism of the lower orders.[59]

## CONCLUSION

In feeling for others and voicing their suffering, the humanitarian narrative, according to Laqueur, tended to create a sense of "property in the objects of compassion."[60] Ownership of property, even in this vein, continued by and large to be the preserve of men, specifically those more learned individuals whose education entitled them to speak on behalf of others. Thus, the degree of sympathy that male professionals could express within the courtroom could sometimes go beyond what any female witness or midwife would dare confess. Some surgeons were quite willing to admit directly their sympathy for the accused, even if it implied a direct disregard for the operations of justice. Dr. Underwood, for instance, testified in Elizabeth Warner's 1770 trial that he had "begged her" when it seemed as if she was "going to say something to me" not to "tell me anything that would do her hurt." Underwood actually advised her at this point to "go away directly," for only she "knew whether she was guilty or not."[61] Such an obvious attempt to obstruct justice as well as such misplaced loyalty—directed as it was toward the accused rather than to abstract principles of truth and objectivity—could not have been made by a female midwife without damage to her reputation. As Laura Gowing maintains, the midwife's position depended on her ability to "expose secrets," specifically those that compromised a community's sexual norms and bodily boundaries.[62] A midwife who testified to having begged a suspect to escape would certainly have jeopardized her role as guardian of female sexual morality. While the purpose of medical evidence was purportedly to establish the facts of the case, the testimony of male midwives and surgeons just as often obscured the "truths" of secret births.

The male medical witnesses in court, while relying upon the dissection of the corpse as a means to interpret the guilt or innocence of the mother, nevertheless frequently utilized their findings in order to make sympathetic and hypothetical claims about the process of delivery and birth. While Rabin maintains that the court's focus upon the state of mind of the defendant became so privileged during the eighteenth century that "evidence about the body no longer determined the outcome of a trial," this statement ignores the way in which the child's body served as the crucial link that allowed medical witnesses to make claims about the intentions of the accused.[63] While women themselves were often the first to draw upon strategies that highlighted their helplessness and vulnerability during delivery—as evidenced by their use of new courtroom defense narratives—it was the corpse itself that was used by medical witnesses, judges, and juries to validate these kind of "confessions."

Unearthing the facts of the case through dissection was vital to these new defenses for reasons other than an ability to offer reliable, scientific truths. As medical testing, such as the floatation of the lungs in water, was increasingly called into question and disallowed as evidence—unless it proved a woman's innocence—by eighteenth-century courts, the evidence available to medical practitioners differed little from that available to traditional midwife witnesses. The testimony offered by these two groups, however, diverged in terms of both the language used and the authority upon which their claims rested. As the experiential knowl-

edge of women came increasingly to be seen as suspect, male practitioners became ever more prominent as expert witnesses in infanticide court
proceedings. The split between innate experiential knowledge and professional objectivity was paralleled by an increasingly articulated division
between communal opinion and educated learning. The shifts occurring
within these trials operated therefore upon an axis of both gender and
class distinctions. The humanitarian narrative, outlined by Laqueur,
worked in some ways as the intersection between these competing
points. Sympathy for the mother as victim exonerated her from guilt
and, simultaneously, helped to affirm the superior feeling and sensibility of the emerging male practitioners and legal professionals. Thus even
while expert medical witnesses confirmed and legitimated women's own
stories of secret births and deliveries, their presence within the proceedings nevertheless called into question women's ability to speak from a
place of authority about their own bodies and the bodies of other
women. As such, while exonerating the accused, the male witnesses also
positioned themselves as the necessary interpreters and narrators of the
female body.

The sympathetic portrayals of accused women within the courtroom
are illustrative of the broader trends surrounding the naturalization and
idealization of motherly love. Through legal practice and medical discourse, a new understanding of motherhood was being created within
the eighteenth-century courtroom.[64] By depicting infanticide as an act
of senseless neglect rather than willful murder, the emergent ideals of
maternal affection could more easily be sustained. Motherhood was
thus both constructed and naturalized through these practices.
Ironically, at the same time that maternal instinct was being expounded
as an innate female sentiment, women's relationship to their own
bodies, to those of other women, and to reproductive knowledge more
generally was increasingly problematized and rendered suspect within
the courtroom. Although maternal instinct was coming to be depicted
as a natural and biologically based female characteristic, this instinct, at
least in cases of secret births, increasingly needed to be mediated by the
(real or symbolic) interposition of the male practitioner. Neither
women's intuitive knowledge nor their innate instincts seemed to be
enough to save the lives of their children during delivery. Women's
helplessness and vulnerability in cases of unattended births thus both
excused them from responsibility and, in some ways, worked to reinforce the claims of male practitioners who argued that women could not
be entrusted with the authority to interpret or manage their own or
other women's bodies.[65]

## NOTES

1. This article is based upon an examination of 187 Old Bailey proceedings for new-born infant murder from 1674 to 1800 (hereafter O.B.P.). The Old Bailey Proceedings Online, Project Directors Tim Hitchcock and Robert Shoemaker, implemented by the Humanities Research Institute, University of Sheffield and the Higher Education Digitization Service, University of Hertfordshire, 2003, www.oldbaileyonline.org (May 15, 2005). During the last quarter of the seventeenth century, records indicate that thirty-five out of the sixty women charged were found guilty, a conviction rate of 58 percent. Beginning in the eighteenth century, fewer cases were being brought to trial and convictions began to decline quite dramatically. From 1700 to 1725 and from 1726 to 1750, 23 percent of women were convicted of the charge, or nine out of thirty-nine and ten out of forty-four respectively. From 1751 to 1775, six out of twenty-nine cases ended in guilty verdicts, a rate of 20.5 percent. During the last quarter of the century, out of a total of fifteen cases, no woman was convicted of the charge. For an examination of conviction rates in other parts of England see, for instance, Peter C. Hoffer and N. E. H. Hull, *Murdering Mothers: Infanticide in England and New England, 1558–1803* (New York: New York University Press, 1981. It should be noted that as of August 1, 2008 the proceedings of the Old Bailey online yields a total of one hundred and ninety-nine cases between 1674 and 1800).

2. The preparation of linen was frequently used as a defense for infanticide in the beginning of this period. The preparation defense involved bringing to court clothes and caps made by the accused for the child in anticipation of its birth. After 1700, this defense was quite successful as it was used to show the court that the accused had every intention of keeping the child should it be born alive.

3. Stephen Landsman, "One Hundred Years of Rectitude: Medical Witnesses at the Old Bailey, 1717-1817," *Law and History Review* 16, no. 3 (Autumn 1998): 445-94, 446.

4. Ibid., 446-47.

5. Ibid., 459. For the advent of increased standards of proof see also Barbara Shapiro, *Beyond 'Reasonable Doubt' and 'Probable Cause': Historical Perspectives on the Anglo-American Law of Evidence* (Berkeley: University of California Press, 1991).

6. Landsman, "One Hundred Years," 447.

7. Ibid., 484.

8. Ibid., 467.

9. 21 James I, c. 27 (1624), *Statutes at Large*, VII, ed. Danby Pickering (Cambridge, 1763), 298, as cited by Hoffer and Hull, *Murdering Mothers*, 20.

10. Jennifer Thorn, "Introduction," in *Writing British Infanticide: Child Murder, Gender and Print, 1722–1859* (Newark: University of Delaware Press, 2003), 13-41, 27.

11. J. M. Beattie, *Crime and the Courts in England, 1660–1800* (Princeton: Princeton University Press, 1986), 113.

12. Hoffer and Hull, *Murdering Mothers*; Mark Jackson, *New-born Child Murder: Women, Illegitimacy and the Courts in Eighteenth-Century England.* (New York: Manchester University Press, 1996); James Kelly, "Infanticide in Eighteenth-Century Ireland," *Irish Economic and Social History* 19, no. 5 (1992): 5–26; R.W. Malcomson, "Infanticide in the Eighteenth Century," in *Crime in England 1550–1800*, ed. J. S. Cockburn (New Jersey: Princeton University Press, 1977).

13. Tracey Rizzo, "Between Dishonour and Death: Infanticide in the Causes Célèbres of Eighteenth-Century France," in *Women's History Review* 13, no. 1 (2004): 5–22, 10. See also, Deborah Symonds, *Weep Not for Me: Women, Ballads, and Infanticide in Early Modern Scotland* (University Park, PA: Pennsylvania State University Press, 1997); Susanne Kord, "Women as Children, Women as Childkillers: Poetic Images of Infanticide in Eighteenth-Century Germany," *Eighteenth Century Studies* 26, no. 3 (Spring 1993): 449–66; Ulinka Rublack, *The Crimes of Women in Early Modern Germany* (New York: Clarendon Press, 1999).

14. Beattie, *Crime and the Courts in England*, 123.

15. Hoffer and Hull, *Murdering Mothers*, 83.

16. Mark Jackson, *New-born Child Murder* (New York: Manchester University Press, 1996), 13.

17. Ibid., 123.

18. Thomas Laqueur, "Bodies, Details, and the Humanitarian Narrative," in *New Cultural History*, ed. Lynn Hunt (Berkeley: University of California Press, 1989), 176–204.

19. The language used by male medical professionals was becoming increasingly specialized and distinct from traditional writings on midwifery. As women were generally denied access to formal scientific training, their language (both written and spoken) remained closer to a more informal and metaphorical style of discourse evident in seventeenth-century manuals. See Ernelle Fife, "Gender and Professionalism in Eighteenth-Century Midwifery," *Women's Writing* 11, no. 2 (2004): 185–200.

20. Dana Rabin, "Bodies of Evidence, States of Mind: Infanticide, Emotion and Sensibility in Eighteenth-Century England," in *Infanticide: Historical Perspectives on Child Murder and Concealment, 1550–2000*, ed. Mark Jackson (Aldershot: Ashgate Publishing Ltd., 2002), 74.

21. O.B.P. Ann Hasle, 1717.

22. O.B.P. Ann Morris, 1722.

23. O.B.P. Ann Gardner, 1708.

24. O.B.P. Mary Gough, 1719.

25. O.B.P. Elizabeth Warner, 1760.

26. I have only counted "droppings" when the accused said (or a witness said on her behalf) that the child dropped from her body during delivery. Most often this was used to explain why the child was found in the vault and/or to explain away bruises and cuts as being merely the result of the child's falling. Being surprised by the onset of labor or being senseless during the time of labor could result in droppings; however, these aspects were not required for this defense to be utilized. Each of these defenses could be used exclusively or in combination.

27. O.B.P. Ann Haywood, 1762.

28. O.B.P. Diana Parker, 1794.

29. O.B.P. Sarah Hunter, 1769.

30. See, for instance, G. J. Barker-Benfield, *The Culture of Sensibility: Sex and Society in Eighteenth-Century Britain* (Chicago: University of Chicago Press, 1992), xix.

31. Landsman, "One Hundred Years," 464-67.

32. Ibid., 465.

33. O.B.P. Ann Taylor, 1779.

34. Roy Porter and Dorothy Porter, *Patient's Progress: Doctors and Doctoring in Eighteenth-Century England* (Cambridge: Polity Press, 1989), 178.

35. Ibid., 178.

36. Jackson, *New-born Child Murder*, 87.

37. Ibid., 87.

38. Ibid., 87.

39. Poisoning, for instance, was another form of murder trial that relied heavily upon autopsy reports and yet one in which the medical evidence presented remained generally inconclusive. See, for example, Ian A. Burney, "Testing Testimony: Toxicology and the Law of Evidence in Early Nineteenth-Century England," *Studies in History and Philosophy of Science* 33 no. 2 (2002): 289-314.

40. Landsman, "One Hundred Years," 455.

41. This trend is also apparent in the fictional representations of infanticide examined by Josephine McDonagh, *Child Murder and British Culture, 1720–1900* (New York: Cambridge University Press, 2003), 32-35.

42. O.B.P. Ann Maybe, 1718.

43. O.B.P. Deborah Greening, 1725.

44. O.B.P. Ann Hullock, 1760. The reference to religion as well as Dorwood's immediate assumption that the accused had committed murder could certainly have

discredited her statement in the eyes of a court increasingly interested in the rules of evidence and scientific experiment. The basis of Dorwood's authority as a woman and midwife rested largely upon experiential knowledge and traditional practice and it was precisely this kind of authority that was increasingly viewed with suspicion in both medical discourse and legal practice. Fife's analysis of the divergent discourses used in male and female midwifery manuals likewise reveals that generally only in women's writing does one find an invocation for God's help toward safe delivery. Fife, "Gender and Professionalism," 186.

45. For a discussion of women's roles as arbiters of bodily boundaries within the community, see Laura Gowing, "Secret Births and Infanticide in Seventeenth-Century England," *Past and Present* 156 (1997): 87–116.

46. O.B.P. Mary Samuel, 1762.

47. That the navel string tore, was cut improperly (without the help of a professional practitioner), or was left untied worked well as a courtroom defense as it played upon the ambiguity of the law with regard to the infant's having a separate identity. By leaving it untied, the effect of the separation between mother and child remained, to a certain degree, incomplete. For a discussion of the symbolic aspects of the navel-string, see Elisabeth Bronfen, "The Body and its Discontents" in *Body Matters: Feminism, Textuality and Corporeality*, ed. Avril Horner and Angela Keane (Manchester: Manchester University Press, 2000).

48. O.B.P. Sarah Hopkins, 1762.

49. O.B.P. Elizabeth Gatskwin, 1779.

50. While female midwives were generally no less sympathetic than male practitioners, the growing preference for "scientific" findings through dissection as opposed to the external evidence traditionally offered by female witnesses gave the male practitioners a larger role in trial proceedings, which seems to have eclipsed what evidence female midwives had to offer.

51. O.B.P. Ann Haywood, 1762.

52. O.B.P. Sarah Russell, 1782.

53. O.B.P. Ann Taylor, 1778.

54. Laqueur, "Bodies, Details," 177.

55. Ibid., 188.

56. O.B.P. Elisabeth Gwatkin, 1779.

57. By making reference to the word of a lady, Mr. Jackson's testimony linked his professionalism with the authority derived from class. A lady's word would obviously have given his opinion more credence than that of unmarried servant women like Gwatkin. Thus, this kind of birth is legitimated not only through the use of scientific discourse, but also through reference to the experiential knowledge of a lady who would, presumably, have no reason to lie.

58. O.B.P. Elizabeth Fletcher, 1749.

59. Tracy Rizzo's examination of infanticide in eighteenth-century French *causes célèbres*, likewise illustrates a growing distrust among judges and juries toward the "bloodlust of the 'peuple'." It was, according to legal authorities, always "misguided public opinion, especially the 'clamor' of women, which created a 'cause célèbre' where none would otherwise exist." Rizzo, "Between Dishonor and Death," 14.

60. Laqueur, "Bodies, Details," 179.

61. O.B.P. Elizabeth Warner, 1770.

62. Laura Gowing, "Ordering the Body: Illegitimacy and Female Authority in Seventeenth-Century England," in *Negotiating Power in Early Modern Society: Order, Hierarchy, and Subordination in Britain and Ireland*, ed. J. M. Braddick and John Walter (Cambridge: Cambridge University Press, 2001), 43–62, 45.

63. Rabin, "Bodies of Evidence," 74.

64. The effects of these shifts have been fairly long-lasting. What had begun in the eighteenth-century as an acceptance on the part of the courts of defenses based on temporary fits of senselessness validated by expert witnesses had, by the nineteenth century, become a medical condition known as puerperal insanity. See, for instance, Hilary Marland, *Dangerous Motherhood: Insanity and Childbirth in Victorian Britain* (New York: Palgrave Macmillan Ltd., 2004).

65. I would like to thank Sara Beam, Andrea McKenzie, and Angus McLaren for their careful reading and helpful suggestions while I was writing the original version of this paper. I also appreciate very much the comments made by Rob Hancock. My research has been supported by a Canada Graduate Scholarships Program Master's Scholarship and the Canadian Graduate Scholarships Program Doctoral Scholarship from the Social Sciences and Humanities Research Council of Canada.

THREE

# "Surely he cannot be flesh and blood"

## The Early Victorian Anatomical Museum and the Blackface Ministrel

STEPHEN JOHNSON

[Juba] married too late (and a white woman besides), and died early and miserably. In a note addressed to Charley White, Juba informed him that, when next he should be seen by Charley, he would be riding in his own carriage. It has been said that in 1852 his skeleton, without the carriage, was on exhibition at the Surrey Music Hall, Sheffield, England.*

—Col. T. Allston Brown, 1877

IN THE LATE SPRING OF 1848 William Henry Lane—whose stage name was "Juba"—a young American dancer of African descent, arrived in London. He appeared as part of a blackface minstrel troupe at Vauxhall Gardens and throughout Britain in the better-class concert halls. Juba received an unusual amount of press. Descriptions of his work ran from rubber-legged

---

*Col. T. Allston Brown, "Among the Minstrels of the Past—The Rise and Fall of Burnt Cork," in *New York Clipper Annals*. From an undated clipping of an end of year retrospective published by the *Clipper*, in the Museum of the City of New York. Internal evidence dates the statement as January 1877 (from reference to the death, one month previously, of minstrel Richard Ward Pelham, whose death registry is dated December 1876).

clown to sublime artist, a "genius of the heels"; his dance was compared to everything from clog, jig, and fling, through whirling dervish and the *wilis* of Romantic ballet, to "the dances of his own simple people on festive occasions." This Juba shone like a bright star in the firmament—of the press, at least—for nearly two years; then, leaving the minstrel troupe, he danced in working-class concert saloons and as a theatrical *entr'acte* hired for the "gallery crowd."[1] He disappeared from documentary view in late 1851 until his reemergence in the statement quoted above, from an early history of minstrelsy, as a skeleton on display in an anatomical museum. This briefly stated, contentious image *embodies* two seemingly disparate phenomena of mid-Victorian popular culture in North America and the United Kingdom—the blackface minstrel show and the anatomical museum.

The case has been made that these two forms rest at opposite ends of a spectrum of cultural performance, the one an exhibition designed to show and teach the absolute control over the body, the other a complete loss of control—the imagining, by turns, of the body in its categorical parts, and the body in its anarchic pieces.[2] On the face of it, this seems an accurate statement. In the event, however, both venues explored common themes by different means: a derogatory depiction of race; the exhibition of the grotesque; and the presentation of the exotic and the (so-called) authentic. In both cases, the body of the "participant" was aggressively manipulated, through the culturally violent removal of flesh and muscle, and the "blacking up" of the minstrel performer. This chapter will briefly examine the ways in which these two forms of display (and of the "show" business) might illuminate each other, and in the process come to an understanding of the strange case noted above: the appearance of one of the most successful performers of his time in his last and longest booking—in a kind of dancer's hell, stripped to the bone and unable to move.

## THE ANATOMICAL MUSEUM

> ...it is to be hoped, that, by seeing the various organs and functions of the human frame, with their varied uses and operations, it will be recollected what miseries may be entailed by a self-willed and wanton destruction of the body.... Many a young person has been saved from vice by an inspection of his Museum....[3]

During the 1840s and 1850s museums of anatomical display became popular as stand-alone commercial attractions. All were similarly structured; Joseph Kahn's and Jacob Reimers's can stand as typical and popular examples. Their catalogues of attractions list hundreds of specimens, a combination of skeletons, wet (preserved in spirits) and dry "preparations," and wax and papier maché models—the distinction between authentic and artificial displays not always clearly delineated. Most items in the exhibition were instructional and developmental: The senses were explained through oversized models; a detailed series of specimens depicted the growth of the fetus; and, more generally, prepared specimens displayed the body in all its parts. Invariably, there were pathological displays depicting what might go wrong with the human anatomy. Some of these illustrated "problems" that were clearly avoidable, the result of the wrongful use and manipulation of the body, as defined by the morality of the exhibitor—the effects of syphilis, smoking, drinking, "onanism" (masturbation), and "the vain fashion of tight lacing in women's dresses." Some specimens presented more "natural" deformities—the conjoined fetus, the skeleton of a giant or a dwarf—though the difference between natural and self-imposed "deformity" was, like the source of the displays, not always clearly distinguished.[4]

The central image of the anatomical museum, whatever other displays and configurations existed, was the figure of the Anatomical Venus, made of wax or, depending on the profile and success of the exhibitor, of papier maché.[5] The gender-segregated audience attended a lecture—man to men, woman to women—in which the functions and placement of all parts of the body were detailed. At first the figure appeared to be a complete naked body of a woman sleeping, typically with one arm raised behind her head. As he spoke, the lecturer would begin to remove the outer layer of the torso, exposing the internal organs. These were then removed, one by one, slowly and with full explanation of place and function. If the catalogue is to be believed, the interior contained at least fourteen separate removable parts.[6] The parts of the body revealed during the lecture were also on display in glass cases to the self-guided visitor; and in both cases, the reclining "anatomical Venus," with the interior exposed, was surrounded by supplementary models and specimens. At every stage, in advertisement and in lecture, two points were emphasized: the aesthetic skill of the artist in the creation of the model, his name advertised at all times, along with the (supposed) classical Greek statuary that served as original; and the pedagogical gifts of the model, which could teach so much more by sight and demonstration than the professional could explain with words. Both points justified, and provided a means of accepting, what might otherwise have been an unnerving experience. Despite this, in the immediate context of the Anatomical Venus, more disquieting and aggressive modes of reception may have been at work. Next to "her," in Reimers's museum, were the following: "the exterior and interior parts of the virgin"; "a perfect specimen of an hermaphrodite who had both sexes united in him...."; "The Consequence of Tight Lacing...; and a "Female Hottentot."...

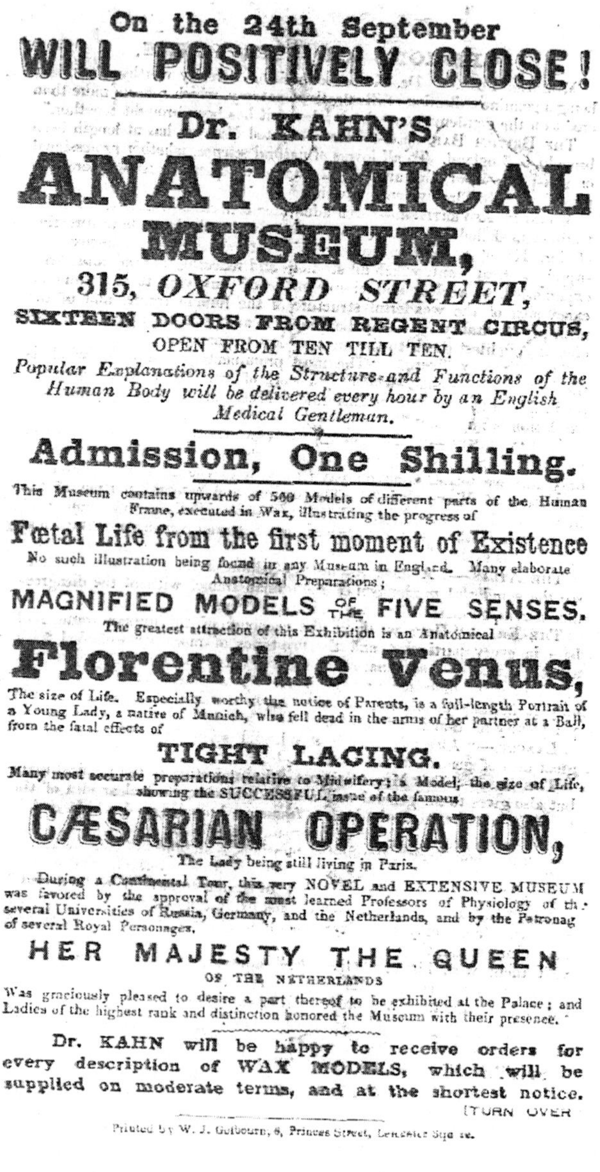

On the 24th September

## WILL POSITIVELY CLOSE!

### Dr. KAHN'S

# ANATOMICAL MUSEUM,

## 315, OXFORD STREET,

### SIXTEEN DOORS FROM REGENT CIRCUS,

OPEN FROM TEN TILL TEN.

*Popular Explanations of the Structure and Functions of the Human Body will be delivered every hour by an English Medical Gentleman.*

## Admission, One Shilling.

This Museum contains upwards of 500 Models of different parts of the Human Frame, executed in Wax, illustrating the progress of

## Fœtal Life from the first moment of Existence

No such illustration being found in any Museum in England. Many elaborate Anatomical Preparations,

## MAGNIFIED MODELS OF THE FIVE SENSES.

The greatest attraction of this Exhibition is an Anatomical

# Florentine Venus,

The size of Life. Especially worthy the notice of Parents, is a full-length Portrait of a Young Lady, a native of Munich, who fell dead in the arms of her partner at a Ball, from the fatal effects of

## TIGHT LACING.

Many most accurate preparations relative to Midwifery; a Model, the size of Life, showing the SUCCESSFUL issue of the famous

# CÆSARIAN OPERATION,

The Lady being still living in Paris.

During a Continental Tour, this very NOVEL and EXTENSIVE MUSEUM was favored by the approval of the most learned Professors of Physiology of the several Universities of Russia, Germany, and the Netherlands, and by the Patronage of several Royal Personages.

## HER MAJESTY THE QUEEN

### OF THE NETHERLANDS

Was graciously pleased to desire a part thereof to be exhibited at the Palace; and Ladies of the highest rank and distinction honored the Museum with their presence.

Dr. KAHN will be happy to receive orders for every description of WAX MODELS, which will be supplied on moderate terms, and at the shortest notice.

[TURN OVER

Printed by W. J. Golbourn, 6, Princes Street, Leicester Square.

**Figure 3.1.** John Johnson Coll. Dr. Khans Anatomical Museum, 1851, Bodleian Library, University of Oxford.

Recent studies of these mid-Victorian museums have emphasized their obsession with both sexuality and race; the early catalogues bear this out. A separate section of the museum typically devoted itself to Embryology, and treated in detail the entire development of the fetus, along with models and specimens, in some numbers, of both male and female sexual organs. Sexually transmitted diseases were given prominence, along with sexual activities considered unorthodox, and developmental deformities. The anatomical museum filled a gap in Victorian society by taking on the role of sex education; both Kahn and Reimers presented lectures on the subject, published pamphlets, and initiated private consultation. The medical profession and the religious status quo by turns praised and criticized this emphasis. To the extent that they framed the explanations as scientific and pedagogical, these museums received generally good press.[7]

Just as common and emphatic in these early museums was the commonly appended "Gallery of All Nations," which presented in diorama form examples of all the "races" of the world, as categorized by the most recent theories of the new science of anthropology. Examples of the great hierarchy of humanity were displayed in wax models–descending from its highest form, the Caucasian, through to the lowest, the "Ethiopian," according to the degree to which the individuals in that branch of the species could control themselves and their environments. A catalogue from Kahn's Museum, printed in 1853, introduces this as a new feature:

> Dr Kahn has also recently added a collection of wax models, taken from life, and exhibiting all the principal varieties of the human race. This collection, which is entirely unrivalled for accuracy, elegance and scientific research, is, moreover, illustrated by popular lectures explanatory of the influences exerted on the human frame by difference of climate, food, and habits of life, together with the modifications caused by peculiarity of temperament, age, and mode of education. Here will be found in one view the graceful Circassian, the angular Copt, the erect European, and the ungainly and ill-poised Ethiopian....[8]

These models served to further emphasize an inherent categorical imperative; within the general hierarchy of race, there were gradations, in the case of the Ethiopian (for example) ranging from "Kaffir Zulus," who "are decidedly superior," through the Hottentots, "the most degraded of which are the Bushmen" (groups of whom were also on display in other venues at this time as living exhibitions), to the "Negro of Nigritia, a specimen of the lowest and most degraded type of the human species." Such displays played out in front of a lay audience the ongoing arguments between proponents of monogenesis, who believed that these were categories of one race altered by environment and life experience, and polygenesis, who proposed that non-Caucasians were entirely separate races.

These pedagogical and aesthetic imperatives provided an overall structure and impetus for anatomical museums, and their goals were aggressively advertised; but it will come as no surprise that a broader range of influences and contexts were also clearly evident. However much it appeared to be organized by rational, categorical principles, the museum took its basic structure from the earlier "cabinet of curiosities" and from exhibitions of "natural" curiosities, which were generally more chaotic and disparate. Whether prepared for public or private consumption, most such collections included many other kinds of items mixed with the anatomical: wax models of events and celebrities, paintings, taxidermy, and any kind of natural objects, all in an idiosyncratic order. Prevalent in such collections were aberrations from any defined norm, pathological or natural. And there were, typically, the trappings and remains of celebrities, notorious or renowned. So, for example, the 1842 inventory for the collection of George Langstaff, a wealthy private collector whose access to "the Workhouse of Cripplegate Parish, the out-poor of a very large district, and my own private practice, have opened to me additional sources," included the "skeleton of a Negro" specifically catalogued, as well as "a sequestrum . . . from the jaw of the late Mr. Joseph Grimaldi, the celebrated clown."[9] The advertisement for Rackstrow's popular touring exhibition of 1782 included:

> An exceeding fine Skeleton of a Woman—They were the bones of Mary Edmonton, who was executed in the year 1759, for the murder of her Aunt, Susanna Walker; A figure of the late Mr. Bamford, the Staffordshire Giant, 7 feet 2 inches high, moulded from him when alive; A Figure of the Late Mr Coan, the Norfolk Dwarf, moulded from him when alive; he was 6 and 30 years of age when he died, measuring 3 feet 6 inches height, and was perfectly straight and well-proportioned.

These identified figures, one "real Preparation" and two "resembling Life," were displayed along with an Egyptian mummy, wax figures of the Royal Family, a rhinoceros hide, and snowshoes from Lapland.[10]

The London catalogue of Reimers's museum betrays the influence of these earlier "cabinets of curiosity." It is difficult to tell, for example, which exhibits are specimens and which are models—that is, which are authentic (or, more correctly, utilize the body itself as the raw material of the preparation) and which are imitations. Some exhibits are completely anonymous (Item 157, "A stomach poisoned from sugar of lead," p. 14), some are located specifically but unnamed (Item 53, "The half-part of a stone extracted from the bladder of an old man in Hull, aged 90, but who died soon after the operation," p. 8), and some are named, with their celebrity detailed. This last category, in particular, includes the natural deformity, particularly models of a "Mr Duval" and "Madame Dimanche," both of whom lived with horn-like growths (Items 164, 165, p. 15). Finally, whether or not intentional, the placement of specimens could be arbitrary, and peculiar: A female skeleton is, for example, located next to "the genitals (penis) of a whale" (Items 125, 126, p. 12).

The Anatomical Museum proliferated during this period as a stand-alone display in part to answer the needs of the medical profession, in two quite different ways. First of all, it was an advocate to the working and lower-middle classes, who were deeply suspicious of the medical profession after decades of grave-robbery scandals, an aversion to the hospital as a kind of institutional incarceration, and a distrust of the very idea of cutting the body in order to cure it. The overall concern was that the body be respected before, during, and after death. The Anatomical Museum attempted to answer that, first of all by creating a reserved, polite, "scientific," and reasonable environment—a place of respect. In this environment, it advocated the empowerment of the individual through self-knowledge: A greater understanding of the parts of the body, the advertisements promised, would lead to a greater understanding and control over the whole. Other lessons were at work, of course. Displays of pathology and deformity emphasized the need to be aware of the potential for disease; the skill of the anatomical artist and the lecturer emphasized the superior knowledge of the medical professional. The presentation of self-inflicted physical deformity emphasized the moral superiority of the anatomist, and the associated displays of natural aberrations reinforced the natural "order" as understood by the profession. In effect, the exhibition of disorder here encouraged a trust in the doctor. "Know thyself," said the advertisements for these museums—but knowledge was not so much power as it was the responsibility to take control over one's body. The body was atomized and categorized—and the individual mind instructed to think of the body in its parts, then to reconstruct it into a manufactured, and thus more manageable, whole. This has been proposed (by Michael Sappol, for example) as constituting a new, anatomical worldview, in which institutional surgery was privileged, but also one in which the body was always thought of from the inside out, in its parts and not as a whole, divided from the mind and controlled by it.

This aggressive emphasis on control betrays a fear of its opposite; a loss of control over the body, and a loss of respect for the body, were legitimate fears at this time for the profession, which had its own internal and external concerns. The culture of the medical student was insular and homosocial. There is evidence that it sanctioned grave robbery—especially of perceived "lesser" races and classes—and made it a practice of initiation. There is also evidence of grotesque manipulation of the body in the privacy of the school, posing corpses in disrespectful and sexually provactive positions. The respect promulgated in the museum, then, could be seen as a teaching aid to the profession itself, as well as to the general public.[11] That public likewise had its own potentially ambivalent attitude toward the body. There was always a visceral, voyeuristic response to these exhibits that could not be completely suppressed by the talk of science and self-control. This is evident in the periodic attacks on anatomical museums by clergymen against the overt display and discussion of sexuality, and their inherent violence.[12] Indeed, the control advocated, even by its supporters, was extreme—as if there was a danger in the anatomical worldview that knowledge of the body might include taking the whole thing apart without putting it back together again.

## MEANWHILE, THE MINSTREL SHOW

Like the anatomical museum, beginning in the 1840s the blackface minstrel "show" became popular as a stand-alone entertainment.[13] As it persisted, prospered, and perhaps ossified, over the next century, it became arguably the most widely disseminated and commercially successful entertainment form of the late nineteenth century. It was still produced by amateurs as recently as the mid-1980s.[14] After the American Civil War it took on a standard set of characteristics familiar to popular memory, including clown-like "endmen" and a stentorian "interlocutor" trading jokes, a prevalence of multipart male harmonies, costumes formulaically alternating between evening wear and "plantation" rustic. In its early, antebellum years, however, such rules did not apply, and anything might have happened on the stage, in any (dis)order. For the sake of this discussion, we can distinguish two characteristics at the core of the phenomenon.

First of all, the fact that a group of men in blackface could carry a full evening's entertainment on their own, without benefit of alternative plot or variety, was itself a surprise; in effect, they set themselves up in opposition to, and as a parody of, an existing touring business of concert-and-variety performers. Later minstrel writing—these performers were very keen to write their own history—expressed a good deal of pride in this ability to compete, and emphasized the hermetic qualities of its society and its skill set. Minstrel performers specialized in that one form for their entire careers, formed fraternities, promulgated "myths" of origin, and moved to increase the respectability, audience, and commercial power of their "industry"—they rated a separate category in lists of touring professionals in the trade papers, co-equal with the "legitimate" touring industry and vaudeville.

At the very core of the form, the one thing all such minstrel events had in common was the consistency of the performer's altered body. This body had an applied black face created from burnt cork mixed with grease; it was consistently black—that is, without shading—and dark to an artificial extreme. This basic makeup was interrupted by red greasepaint around the mouth, creating the appearance of artificially large lips. On top of the head was a wig of short, curly black "hair." Costuming varied widely, but can generally be characterized as rustic and distressed, with rips and patches, or as garish and urban, ill-fitting and with bold mismatched colors. There was a strong tendency toward the accessorizing we now associate with the clown, in particular oversized shoes and collars (into which the head could disappear on cue), and striped pants or stockings at odds with the rest of the costuming. To all of this might be added specialty costuming, especially for the near-universal "wench" dance, in which a cross-dressed performer was serenaded.

Singing and dancing was what this body did on stage. The instruments included the very new banjo, advertised as an African and southern slave invention; but it was always accompanied by the tambourine (more like the Irish folk *bourrín*), and the "bones," a variation on the "spoons" or castanets. These three core instruments emphasized percussion, improvisation, and unusual, syncopated rhythmic variations; they were played, by all accounts, with a whole-body passion, the blacked-up masked figures frenetically jerking and adopting unusual stances as if barely able to keep their seats, interrupting these with sudden and quite artificial slow and stately rhythm and movement. To this core beat was added, typically, a fiddle and (less often, but surprisingly) the accordian as melodic instruments. The common image of the minstrel show that persists today begins and ends with the performance of a number of dialect standards—Buffalo Gals, Camptown Races, and Oh Susanna. These songs were certainly standard features, and the sheet music for them a major source of income for publishers and (at least indirectly) performers; but we might better think of them as the stimuli for a highly energized, possibly exhausting evening of near-chaos. So it was described, at least. The following focuses on Gilbert Pell, the bones of the Ethiopian Serenaders in 1848:

> FREE-TRADE HALL.—"Juba" and the Serenaders.—A party of serenaders, under the leadership of Mr. G. W. Pell, late of St. James's Theatre, gave one of their peculiar exhibitions on Monday evening in the Free-trade Hall. They are six in number, and are mostly happy in the possession of nigger-like physiognomies. The "making up" of their leader was

extremely ludicrous. With literally a yard of shirt collar and frill, it was scarcely possible to witness his extravagant grimaces, without a most undignified unbending of the facial muscles, and many were the handkerchiefs employed to conceal the smothered laughter of their fair owners.[15]

The minstrels, seated (barely) in a rough semi-circle, ranged from jokes based on the bad pun, through parodies of classical operatic music and dance styles, burlesques of well-known plots (often Shakespeare or the opera), and so-called stump speeches, parodying contemporary events, trends, and politics through a mock-stentorian speech in the malaprop-prone dialect common to all minstrel performers (and still recognizable to us today, so persistent was its influence).

The unusual character of the early minstrel show—and its distance from our own sensibilities or common misperceptions of it—can be summed up in its two most popular early numbers. The first was the Railroad Overture, in which the entire troupe, using every instrument and voice, and every part of every body in motion and sound, imitated that new, revolutionary, and noisy transportation technology. The second was the wench dance Lucy Long, in which a young white male in black-face and a comic drag costume purported to approximate a southern slave wearing her mistress' mismatched hand-me-downs, danced by turns in a slow walk-around and an out-of-control "breakdown" to a grotesque (and violent) song of praise ("Oh, she's a lubly creature, Tho' her mouth is rather wide"):

> And if she prove a scolding wife,
> I'll whip her sure yer born,
> And I'll take her down to New Orleans
> And sell her off for corn![16]

This was sung to "her" by other young white men in blackface—the whole advertised as an authentic re-creation of Southern plantation culture. Here, in both cases, were images of an artificially created body, out of control, and yet in imitation.

On its face, minstrelsy was advertised as imitation—hence the common epithet "Ethiopian Delineators"—specifically of Southern plantation slave culture. We will return to the reasons for this claim; but recent writing on the subject has made it clear that the sources and contexts for this phenomenon ranged more widely.[17] Some scholars have stressed potential folk and ritual sources, which can be difficult to prove but are evocative nonetheless: the existence of a folk character among Southern black Americans called "Jim Crow," a trickster figure with roots in Africa; Western European traditions of charivari and carnival, which included

# THEATRE ROYAL, BIRMINGHAM.
# PELL'S SERENADERS
AND
# BOZ's JUBA
☞ POSITIVELY THE LAST 2 NIGHTS. ☜
## THIS EVENING, THURSDAY, DEC. 21, 1848,
# BENEFIT OF BOZ'S JUBA.
## TO-MORROW EVENING, FRIDAY,
# BENEFIT OF G. W. PELL

The Nobility, Gentry, and Public in general are respectfully informed, that the above are positively THE ONLY NIGHTS this EXTRAORDINARY COMPANY can perform in Birmingham, as they commence in Wolverhampton on Saturday, the 23rd.

## CHANGE OF PROGRAMME
### NEW SONGS, GLEES, REFRAINS, CHANTS, OVERTURES, &c. &c. &c.
#### PART FIRST.

OVERTURE,..................................................................................................BAND.
GLEE—" You'll see dem on de Ohio,"..............................................................COMPANY.
CHANT—" I seen her at de Window,".......................................................................PELL.
BALLAD—" Darkies, lament,".................................................................................IRWIN.
SONG—" Ladies, won't you marry ?".................................................................VALINTINE.
SONG—" Floating Scow,"....................................................................................LUDLOW.
SOLO AND CHORUS—" Stop dat Knockin !".............................VALINTINE AND COMPANY.

## "MISS LUCY LONG," IN CHARACTER, (ORIGINAL,) - BOZ'S JUBA.

*INTERVAL OF FIVE MINUTES.*

#### PART SECOND.

OVERTURE,..................................................................................................BAND.
SONG—" My Skiff is by de Shore,".........................................................................IRWIN.
SONG—" Ohio Boatman,".................................................................................VALINTINE.
CHANT—" Railroad Travelling,"...............................................................................PELL.
REFRAIN—" Picayune Butler,"..............................................................................IRWIN.
BALLAD—" Mary Blane,"...............................................................................VALINTINE.
CHANT—" My Old Aunt Sally,"...............................................................................IRWIN.

*INTERVAL OF FIVE MINUTES.*

#### PART THIRD.

OVERTURE,..................................................................................................BAND.
SOLO AND CHORUS—" Come with a Darkey Band,"......................VALINTINE AND COMPANY.
CHANT—" Dandy Broadway Swell,"..........................................................................IRWIN.
REFRAIN—" Come back, Stephen,".............................................................................JUBA.
SONG—" Sambo's Ghost,".......................................................................................IRWIN.
CHANT—" Jenny, put de Kittle on,"............................................................................JUBA.

## FESTIVAL DANCE, (ORIGINAL,)   -   -   -   BOZ'S JUBA.
## PLANTATION DANCE, (ORIGINAL,)   -   -   -   BOZ'S JUBA.
### ACCOMPANIED ON THE BANJO BY BRIGGS, THE BEST PLAYER IN THE WORLD.

☞ Mr. PELL would take it as a great Favour if the Audience would withhold their Applause until the end of MASTER JUBA'S Dances ; by doing so, they will hear the *exact* Time he keeps with his EXTRAORDINARY STEPS.

**LOWER BOXES, 3s.——UPPER BOXES, 2s.——PIT, 1s.——GALLERY, 6d.**
HALF-PRICE TO THE BOXES AT THE END OF THE SECOND PART.
Doors to be opened at Half-past Seven o'Clock ; the Performance will commence at Eight. Carriages at a Quarter past Ten.
**The Box-Office is open Daily, from Eleven till Three, where Tickets and Places may be secured. Box Book-keeper, Mr. YATES.**

FREDERICK TURNER, PRINTER, SNOWHILL.

**Figure 3.2.** Playbill for the Ethiopian Serenaders with Juba. Note how Juba is separated from the group typographically and as a part of bill structure, yet he is also included as part of the troupe. Birmingham Central Library.

blacked-up devil figures, some also cross-dressed; and even proposed con-nections with the tradition of Harlequin—another trickster in a black mask, a patchwork costume and a strong dialect. Others have proposed that the early minstrel show represented an effort by show business entre-preneurs to capture and tame a vibrant, uniquely diverse street culture.

By this scenario, there existed in the port and waterway cities of the United States (and the Atlantic more generally) a chaotic, hybridized cul-ture consisting of the languages, songs, dances, and humor of a full range of northern European and Mediterranean immigrant cultures, commin-gling in the out-of-doors working world of barges and ships, and the sea-port world of dance halls, saloons, brothels, and tenements. Into this mix, during the first half of the nineteenth century, came a large influx of freed and runaway slaves from the Southern states, whose culture tended to co-opt and be co-opted by the European cultures. Thus percussive clog, jig, and flamenco dance from Ireland, Lancashire, and Spain commingled with a very different aesthetic from western Africa, and English folk-song with syncopation. A description (and illustration) of a dance competition on the streets of Boston is revelatory:

> The first dance on the list was a hornpipe, and the one who took the most steps was to come off victor. It was Bryant's first turn, and as she entered the ring, she made three courtesies to the spectators who formed three sides about her. The word was given; the negro fiddler struck up Fisher's Hornpipe, and Susan commenced—and the way she put in the big licks was a "sin to Moses."[18]

The competition includes minstrel-like songs, a black fiddler, women as competitors, and a thoroughly mixed-race and (perhaps) mixed-class specta-torship. The description of the dancers defines the loss of control and the (inappropriate) display of the body in public. This popular, chaotic sensi-bility can be seen as a primary source for the minstrel show, which was, however, not imitated without alteration.

The "show business" of the nineteenth century—that is, the culture that created commodity capital out of exhibition and performance—not surprisingly co-opted this thriving street culture, first of all to attract paying customers from the working classes into their venues.[19] Those features of the blackface minstrel described above that appear clown-like can be traced to this character's common appearance in the circus for decades prior to the minstrel show, as a kind of rustic figure that, again not surprisingly, combined song, dance, acrobatics, and "patter" in many combinations. Such performers were also common in the variety saloons of the period, venues that were, quite unlike the minstrel shows, racially and gender-inte-grated on stage, if not in the audience.

Their presence, in their early incarnations, appeared to be more immediately politicized than other kinds of performers. George Washington Dixon, for example, combined a political career with that of a blackface performer and comic, presenting his nativist, anti-immigration, and class-conscious messages as stump speeches, on stage and in the local press. Thomas Dartmouth Rice, who had a truly astonishing career from the 1830s, used the character of "Jim Crow" to sing an ever-changing round of political and social satire.[20] Eric Lott, in *Love and Theft*, depicts a complex relationship between performer and audience—particularly working-class white male audiences—that remained significant during the early years of the minstrel show. His picture is ambivalent in the extreme, at once racially motivated and demeaning toward freedmen and runaways, mocking their incompetence at anything ostensibly civilized—fashion, dance, song, language, and understanding. It was in this sense meant to bind the audience in a position of superiority, the black body standing in for any immigrant group, for women, for any "other." On the other hand, in the early days of the use of the term "wage slave," the laboring classes could identify both with any depiction of a powerless culture and with the backhanded mockery toward the middle classes generated from having an "inferior" character imitate it "badly." The white performer used the role of the black trickster to mock everyone's "betters"; and it was by all accounts attractive to those first male audiences. Anarchy, apparently, was encouraged. The blackface clown resonated—out of control, angrily inept, and unable to fit into a "white" society in lyric, choreography, and narrative.

Show business has always prospered by co-opting popular street culture for profit, but it also abhors chaos. It is always already, even as it imitates, creating repeatable formulae that will allow it to reproduce and disseminate its product as widely as possible geographically and to as broad an audience as possible. The commercial needs of the early minstrel show of necessity altered its most immediate roots, controlling and curtailing those elements that would drive away the middle classes, as well as women and children and all other paying customers. The means by which they did so—through manipulations of race, class and gender—are more easily delineated (like "Ethiopians") by analogy to its contemporary and contiguous exhibition form, the anatomical museum. Slavery, combined with life in the Deep South, makes a person an "Ethiopian" in the "Gallery of All Nations," and "black," by this scenario, is equated with the deformity manifested in the minstrel show caricature.

The emphasis on the minstrel body's proximity to an original, and the distance of the artist from that original, reinforced a greater consistency and control over the performance than could be argued for a folk or street culture, a circus performer, or a political satirist. The body on stage by this argument only *seemed* out of control. Through the exhibition of clearly rehearsed and controlled performance, the enjoyment of these bodies in motion was in fact the result of the training and artistry of white men. The delineation of these characters *exhibited* the body out of control, and its results. Like the anatomical museum, it conflated and confused intentional and "natural" abnormality, and presented race as "naturally" inferior, incapable of either grace or morality in the world. The lesson by negative example was, like that of the anatomical museum, that the means to self-improvement was greater control over the body.

## JUBA ON THE MINSTREL STAGE

"[Juba] jumps, he capers, he crosses his legs, he stamps his heels, he dances on his knees, on his ankles, he ties his limbs into double knots...."[21] The essential defining image of minstrelsy was that of a white man, through artifice, creating a controlled aesthetic image of a "natural" absence of control—physical and vocal as well as intellectual and ethical. If Juba was performing with the same kind of wild abandon, he was doing so without the aesthetic controlling mechanism; he was, instead, "authentically" out of control. This seems to suggest that he would be a dangerous figure on stage, and surely viewed as an exception to the rules of that stage—unless there were alternative controlling strategies. With the lessons of the anatomical and ethnographic museum in mind, certain characteristics of the reviews and advertisements for this entertainer do stand out.

The problem of Juba's authenticity was played out in reviews and advertisements as part of his attraction. He was described more often and in greater detail than any other minstrel performer; writers competed in their attempts to describe his dance, and typically (and rhetorically) admitted their failure to do so. These descriptions careened from a vision of complete chaos to absolute control, combining images of impossible contortions of legs and arms with rhapsodizing about the precise control over his tapping and choreography. Following are just two examples:

> His pedal execution is a thing to wonder at, if his flexibility of muscle did not confound us. He jumps, he capers, he crosses his legs, he stamps his heels, he dances on his knees, on his ankles, he ties his limbs into double knots, and untwists them as one might a skein of silk, and all these marvels are done in strict time and appropriate rhythm—each note has its corresponding step and action. Now he languishes, now burns, now love seems to sway his motions, and anon rage seems to impel his steps. Juba's

plantation dance is a sort of terpsichorean illustration of Collin's "Ode on the Passions."[22]

> Surely he cannot be flesh and blood, but some more subtle substance, or how could he turn, and twine, and twist, and twirl, and hop, and jump, and kick, and throw his feet almost with a velocity that makes one think they are playing hide-and-seek with a flash of lightning! Heels or toes, on feet or on knees, on the ground or off, it is all the same to Juba; his limbs move as if they were stuffed with electric wires....[23]

We might read into this reaction a kind of distress with the image that was being worked out in the writing. It is likely that the invitation to describe him—and therefore to proscribe him—was part of the publicity campaign for his tour.[24]

In places, reviewers used an almost ethnographic detail in their descriptions of his dance:

> He is apparently about eighteen years of age; about 5 feet 3 inches in height; of slender make, yet possessing great muscular activity. His head is very small, and his countenance, when at rest, has a rather mild, sedate, and far from unpleasing expression....[25]

as if he was something other than a minstrel performer, not there for his entertainment value or the exhibition of his skill, but as an object for close study. Advertisements, although including him as a member of the troupe, habitually included a contiguous advertisement for Juba alone, as if his performance was a separate event embedded within the evening's minstrel show. Playbills were similarly organized, in boldface advertising Juba's entry and solo—as if he then left the stage to the "real," that is to say "false," minstrels.

While with the minstrel show—and, tellingly, not in any other venue—Juba performed the wench dance, cross-dressed as Miss Lucy Long. As described above, this standard of early minstrelsy involved a performer in a garish, mismatched dress, dancing to a song by one or more of the other minstrels:

> Juba makes his appearance on the stage attired in the habiliments of a stylish lady: pink muslin dress, blue bonnet, green parasol and, as a kind of foundation to this gaudy gear, a pair of red morocco boots. Juba is accompanied by Pell, suitably equipped as a Broadway dandy; this latter sits and sings to the accompaniment of the banjo, violin, and tambourine, the well-known ditty of "Lucy Long," while Juba is executing the

most difficult pas, introducing double-shuffles, pirouettes, and every imaginary step to be achieved by the nimble foot.[26]

It is difficult to justify this portrayal, for which there is no evidence that he used the blackface makeup. We are left with the ambivalent image of a young black male, not in blackface, in a dress, dancing by turns in a slow drag and a fast breakdown, all to the singing of young white men in blackface. In the playbills, this dance appears to be presented as yet another "authentic" solo, though it was neither. The implied authenticity might have been a defense for what was certainly a unique sight for an audience—a black man in a dress.

Negative comments began to creep into the references to Juba after he left the minstrel troupe and returned to the (more integrated) variety houses and saloons of the working classes. He was admonished not to "jump too fast," and his attractions were all labelled as attractive only to the "rougher" and "less refined" members of the audience. Without the context of the minstrel show, this performer's skill-set appears to have become unacceptable—out of control. Or, alternatively, he changed his dance.[27]

## JUBA AT THE ANATOMICAL MUSEUM

"[Juba] was married … to a white woman, lived a fast life, dissipated freely, and died miserably during the season of 1851–2. It has been stated that his skeleton was on exhibition at the Surrey Music Hall, Sheffield, Eng."[28] The similarities embedded in these seemingly disparate forms—the minstrel show and the anatomical museum—are thrown into relief by, and in turn help to explain, the presence of Juba. In microhistorical terms William Henry Lane was an "exceptional normal," that is, a phenomenon that is taken as normal in its original context and yet appears exceptional to contemporary eyes.[29] Lane/Juba was a performer of color, the only one present in early blackface minstrelsy. He appeared without blackface, apparently as a fully accepted member of the troupe.[30] This fact clearly flies in the face of the standard features of the minstrel form and also of the control mechanisms described above. How could this be, and how could he be accepted on stage? Why would his body move from minstrel show to museum, and was this an aberration because he himself was an aberration—or was it entirely appropriate to the relationship between the two forms? Having established a connection between the mid-nineteenth-century anatomical museum and the blackface minstrel show, stimulated by reference to the appearance of a minstrel performer in an anatomical museum, three questions need to be addressed. The first is whether the specific reference to

Juba as an anatomical specimen holds any merit as fact. The second is what place that performer would have had in such an appearance. The third is what this "report" can tell us "in any event."

The answer to the first question is that, while debatable, it is probable that the Juba reference is correct, the evidence circumstantial but persuasive. The description of Lane—"Boz's Juba"—on display first appears in a lengthy obituary of another performer who had just died in Liverpool in 1876, and was written by T. Allston Brown, a long-time booking agent, writer, and editor for the show-business trade journal *The New York Clipper*—a well-known collector of theatrical memorabilia. It is repeated, with some variation of prose, in a 1912 history of minstrelsy published in the same paper. Brown's ongoing contributions of old programs, odd items, and thumbnail sketches of life on the road, published over forty years in the *Clipper*, are a treasure trove for historians, but they have also proven themselves surprisingly accurate whenever corroboration exists.[31] In other words—at odds with the amateur nature of the collecting and the itinerant nature of the subject matter—Brown was a reliable historian. This appears to be the case in the reference to Juba. He did indeed disappear from the record late in 1851, after regular reports of performances throughout Britain.

Second, Juba was presented in the minstrel show as both a celebrity and a natural curiosity. He was famous as himself, and not as a masked figure portraying something other than himself. As such he fell into the category shared by "Mr. Coan the Norfolk Dwarf," or "Mary Edmonton, executed...for the murder of her aunt" (see the description above), and other exhibitions postmortem of the abnormal—that abnormality confusing, as it habitually did, the physiological and the moral. Juba was famous, and preternaturally, indescribably, abnormally talented, and as such his presence tapped into the vestiges of the fairground exhibition and the cabinet of curiosities still evident in midcentury museums. Reinforcing his presence here is the matter of race, which during this period had become a major exhibition strategy in the anatomical museum, depicting difference through both authentic and fabricated specimens, in the form of cranial and skeletal measurements, size and weight, cultural and environmental circumstances. Unlike his masked fellow performers, Juba's skeleton (at least), specifically named or anonymously (and typologically) racialized, would have multiple uses in the anatomical museum as an embodiment of race, of celebrity, and of abnormality.

The third, and easily the most important point to be raised, is what we might learn about the culture of that time and place from the Brown reference. When he ties the two forms of exhibition together, Brown does so as the moral tale of a man who is suitably punished for a number of clearly delineated reasons—for miscegenation, for arrogance, for rising above his "natural" station as an inferior being, and for losing control of his body, finally, in a vaguely articulated dissolute existence. In this moral tale, the body of Juba becomes the minstrel performer's worst nightmare—to be misrepresented as black, as authentic, as out of control, and thus misjudged as inferior. This attitude toward Juba's body, as it might be "punished" by display, resonates throughout the other evidence of that body's existence in life—and in the minstrel show.

## CONCLUSION

I believe all of these observations suggest a set of controls over Juba's dancing body, and a reason for his presence on the otherwise strictly segregated minstrel stage. In effect, he was not a part of the minstrel performance but "on exhibition" along with that performance, just as surely as bodies depicting race, gender, and class were on exhibition in the anatomical museum. He was as aggressively advertised as an authentic Southern slave (a doubtful claim), "being" and not "acting."[32] Audiences were encouraged through the descriptions both to examine him in a precise categorical manner and to negotiate with language to lay claim to his choreography. His cross-dressing, as strange as it may seem, may have served as a distraction from his presence as an authentic racial body. It may also have provided an aggressive and obvious physical control over his dance. And, by identifying his race with the feminine, it may have served to curtail his no doubt considerable sexual attraction.[33] The result of all of these controlling mechanisms, both subtle and obvious, was to create an exhibition of authenticity in the midst of a stage filled with artifice. Like the skeleton and the prepared tissues surrounding the wax models of the anatomical museum, he was there to provide authenticity-by-association. When he left the minstrel show, without that frame, he could no longer be controlled.

There is one last image from which a more complex understanding of Juba might be generated, and that itself provides a bridge between the minstrel show and the anatomical museum. On one of the advertisements for the performances by the Ethiopian Serenaders at Vauxhall Gardens, there is a portrait of Juba that is a finely detailed work, clearly taken from a daguerrotype. This is unusual for the year, 1848, and doubly significant as an early image of a black entertainer. At first glance it seems a respectful homage and a sign of importance within the industry—but not in the light of this discussion. The other image in this advertisement is G. W. Pell, whose representation is not from a daguerrotype, nor is it particularly detailed. It is not unreasonable to think that one daguerrotype deserved another, unless there was a different reason for its existence. The early minstrel performers were insistent that their images as white entertainers be depicted on sheet music, if not playbills, as well as the images of their characters as minstrels; it was important that they be perceived first as white, then as skilled. Pell's image exists in this advertisement to emphasize just such a generic "white-

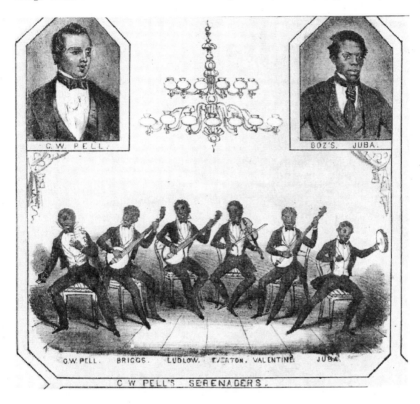

**Figure 3.3.** Illustration of the 1848 version of the Ethiopian Serenaders at Vauxhall Gardens, from a poster. In the depiction of the troupe, Juba appears as the "tambo." Above, his image is taken from a daguerrotype, in contrast to the more generic representation of Pell (the other "endman" or "bones"). The Harvard Theatre Collection, Houghton Library.

ness"; Juba's image, by contrast, exists to advertise his specific "blackness." The message of this portrait is not simply that he belongs to another race; another image of him serves that purpose more appropriately, giving him a "stock" minstrel head. The daguerrotype reinforces the idea that race is embedded in his character. It serves the opposite function to Pell's portrait, clearly stating that Juba's body is not "fabricated." This is both his attraction

and his danger. In the later years of minstrelsy, such authenticity was controlled in other ways—performers of color blacked up in order to perform,
controlling their alleged authenticity through complete erasure. The chaotic
early days of minstrelsy were not so efficient.

If I were to go further down this slippery exegetical slope, I would
draw attention to the physical process of creating a daguerrotype. Roland
Barthes draws the connection in *Camera Lucida*:

> Photography transformed subject into object, and even, one might say,
> into a museum object: in order to take the first portraits...the subject
> had to assume long poses under a glass roof in bright sunlight; to become
> an object made one suffer as much as a surgical operation; then a device
> was invented...which supported and maintained the body in its passage
> to immobility....[T]his headrest was the pedestal of the statue I would
> become....

He adds: "Death is the eidos of that Photograph."[34] In this passage, Barthes
finds a similarity among the process and product of early photography, the
museum exhibition, and the medical procedure. They are all instances of
the body under conditions of extreme control, to which this chapter argues
we may add the minstrel show—however backhanded the presentation of
the controlling culture. When Allston Brown made the anatomical display
of Juba his punishment for rising above his station—believing himself a
celebrity of importance, marrying a white woman, bragging—he was only
taking to the anatomical extreme the variety of ongoing efforts to gain control over that body through the minstrel show and the museum.

## NOTES

1. The history of Juba has been compiled from a review of numerous contemporary
   periodicals and incorporated into a database and Web site. See
   http://link.library.utoronto.ca/minstrels/. For "genius of his heels," see *Theatre
   Journal*, August 1, 1850, p. 347, col. 2 for reference to whirling dervishes and
   the wilis, see *Era*, June 18, 1848, p. 13, col. 1 for "dances of his own simple
   people," see *Manchester Guardian*, October 18, 1848 p. 5, col. 4 for "gallery
   crowd" see the *Huddersfield Chronicle and West Yorkshire Advertiser*, November
   30, 1850, p. 5, col. 1.

2. I am indebted specifically to Michael Sappol's work on the nineteenth-century
   anatomical museum for the idea of the minstrel as a body out of control in a
   society for which this was both captivating and troublesome. Michael Sappol, *A
   Traffic in Dead Bodies: Anatomy and Embodied Social Identity in Nineteenth-
   Century America* (Princeton: Princeton University Press, 2002). He in turn cites

Eric Lott, *Love and Theft : Blackface Minstrelsy and the American Working Class* (New York: Oxford University Press, 1993).

3. From a catalogue of J.W. Reimers, *J. W. Reimers's Gallery of All Nations and Anatomical Museum* (London,1853).

4. The crucial works on the nineteenth-century anatomical museum are Michael Sappol, *A Traffic in Dead Bodies*, focusing on the United States; Maritha Rene Burmeister, "Popular Anatomical Museums in Nineteenth-Century England," Dissertation (State University of New Jersey, New Brunswick/Rutgers, 2000); and Ruth Richardson, *Death, Dissection and the Destitute* (London: Routledge and Kegan Paul, 1987). All three corroborate the complex class conflict surrounding the corpse and the museum during these years. The influences of Foucault, Butler, and Gramsci are clearly behind these works, particularly Sappol; and, more generally, Merleau-Ponty's statement that "The body is an historical idea" in *The Phenomenology of Perception*, trans. Colin Smith (Boston: Routledge and Kegan Paul, 1962). On the body, science, race, sexuality, and the museum, see Tony Bennett, *The Birth of the Museum: History, Theory, Politics* (London: Routledge, 1995), Martin Kemp and Marina Wallace, *Spectacular Bodies: The Art and Science of the Human Body from Leonardo to Now* (Berkeley: University of California Press, 2000), and Ludmilla Jordanova, *Sexual Visions: Images of Gender in Science and Medicine between the Eighteenth and Twentieth Centuries* (New York: Harvester Wheatsheaf, 1989). On race, science, and exhibition see, Jane Goodall, *Performance and Evolution in the Age of Darwin: Out of the Natural Order* ( London: Routledge, 2002), Nancy Stepan, *The Idea of Race in Science: Great Britain, 1800–1960* (London: Archon Books, 1982), Lernth Lindfors, ed., *Africans on Stage: Studies in Ethnological Show Business* (Bloomington: Indiana University Press, 1999), and especially Sander L. Gilman, *Difference and Pathology: Stereotypes of Sexuality, Race and Madness* (Ithaca: Cornell University Press, 1985). A range of playbills and catalogues examined for this chapter is located in the John Johnson Collection, Bodleian Library, Oxford University, the Wellcome Library for the History of Medicine, and the British Library. In particular: Joseph Kahn, *Catalogue of Dr. Kahn's Anatomical Museum* (London, 1851), which lists and describes 341 items, and J.W. Reimers, *J. W. Reimers's Gallery of All Nations and Anatomical Museum* (Leeds, 1853), which lists 410 and claims more than 450 items on display. For information, see illustrations, and the following sample "tour" published in the *Era*, March 30, 1851:

> DR. KAHN'S ANATOMICAL EXHIBITION—To be understood by the general reader, for whom we write (more than we do for the professional man, who must look elsewhere for the technicalities which alone can give a minute description of that to which are about to refer), we must simply state that Dr. Kahn, a German surgeon, well known in his own country, has opened to the public, at 315, Oxford-street, an exhibition, perhaps the most extraordinary which, at this time, invites inspection, and what he terms an "*Anatomical Museum*." This is, in fact, a collection which has

occupied his time for many years past, and one which exhibits more of poor human nature than we should like to describe, were we ever so capable of undertaking the task. We see preparations from life, and others of what once belonged to life itself, models in leather, casts in wax, realities so carefully preserved, similitudes so striking, imitations so exquisite, and illustrations so perfect, that the mind is bewildered by the reflections they suggest, and the truths they reveal. Here we have the economy of the human frame laid bare in every particular, and the mysteries of mortality unfolded with artistic skill and minute precision, at once a curious and an edifying sight. We see anatomical figures taken to pieces bit by bit, and the process of digestion explained. We behold large models of the eye and the ear, and strange degrees of comparison. A lecturer attends, and with his subject literally at his fingers' ends, explains, with remarkable ease and perspicuity, all that is before you. You have particular organs and functions cleverly described, structures so finely moulded that you cannot help admiring the ingenuity of man, even while you see the surprising workmanship of his Maker. Arteries, veins, and muscles, are represented plainly and accurately. But a series of figures exhibiting the progress of a human being, from the earliest origin that can be perceived, to maturity is of itself a remarkable collection of figures, and here they are, for the lovers of science and the explorer of nature. We see what tight lacing will do, and what more reprehensible acts will bring to pass—"a sorry sight!" The visitor, however, must not imagine that he goes to explore an exhibition similar to that of Madame Tussaud's. These are works of art—subjects for philosophical contemplation. Having overcome a natural repugnance, you examine what you see for the sake of the knowledge to be gathered, and you come away with mingled humiliation and awe—a profitable impression. Something of this kind has been for many years exhibited at Paris, but the whole museum may be regarded as a novelty. Artists of no mean ability have been employed in the construction of these illustrations of what exists, but few know anything about. We will not be more exact in our details, but we wish it to be understood that the museum is well worthy the inspection of both the professional and non-professional man. It will afford amusement to the merely curious, and astonish the most stolid, for these revelations go home, and, in looking upon what we see, we are unavoidably reminded of the common laws which regulate the formation of peer and peasant-lady and scullery-maid."

5. This figure was sometimes called the Florentine Venus; there was also an "Anatomical Adonis," though this model was not as prevalent, according to my own research. The museum display was revolutionized by the development of the papier maché models of Louis Auzoux. See Mark Dreyfuss, "The Anatomical Models of Dr. Auzoux," in *Medical Heritage* 2, no. 1 (January-February 1986): 60-62. Further material related to Auzoux was examined in the British Library.

6. From Reimers (London, 1853), 26: Larynx, Scutiforme cartilage, Windpipe, Ascending blood-vessel, Descending blood-vessel, Lungs, Heart spit, Heart, Midriff, Liver, Stomach, Bowels, Caul, Bladder.

7. For reference, from a bill advertising "Dr. Kahn's Museum and Gallery of Science," 1858:

"Opinions of the press on Dr. Kahn's anatomical collection:
Lancet: Altogether, it is a splendid scientific collection; and a great deal of general information is to be obtained by a visit.
The Medical Times: The Museum is decidedly the best ever exhibited in London; and we recommend our readers to pay Dr. Kahn a visit.
Weekly Chronicle: If such exhibitions as that of Dr. Kahn's were calculated only to gratify the morbid curiosity of a vulgar and unthinking mind, they would indeed be to little purpose; but to such as visit them with higher motives, and a humble desire to witness the Divine power in some of His most marvellous, most minute, and most elaborate works, they will prove both elevating and instructive.
Morning Advertiser: . . . it supplies a great art, which all studious and reflecting persons must have experienced, of a clear and simple mode of conveying to the mind an exact idea of the wonderful structure of the human frame, and of the principle of vitality. It may be proper to add, that no object in it will offer the slightest shock to the most modest temperament.

8. Joseph Kahn, Catalogue of Doctor Kahn's Anatomical Museum, now exhibiting at the Portland Gallery, 316 Regent Street, opposite the Polytechnic Institution (London, n.d.). In the British Library, iv; subsequent quotations are from the section titled "Gallery of All Nations—Ethiopian Variety," 26–27. The exhibition of race and the exotic in this period was widespread. See Richard Altick, The Shows of London (London: Belknap Press, 1978), among a range of more recent writing. More specifically, the Morning Chronicle (May 27, 1846) advertises the Ethiopian Serenaders in the same column as the exhibition of a Maori chieftain and Scottish dwarves. The Observer (May 2, 1847) advertises the exhibition of South African Aborigines or Bushmen. Such displays were numerous, and included, at least as advertised, a group of African Americans.

9. From George Langstaff, Catalogue of the Preparations illustrative of Normal, Abnormal, and Morbid Structure, Human and Comparative, constituting the Anatomical Museum of George Langstaff (London: John Churchill, 1842).

10. From Benjamin Rackstrow, A descriptive catalogue (giving a full explanation) of Rackstrow's Museum: consisting of a large, and very valuable collection of most curious Anatomical Figures, and real Preparations; also Figures resembling Life; with a great variety of Natural and Artificial Curiosities; to be seen at No. 197 Fleet-Street, between Chancery-Lane and Temple Bar (London, 1782), in the Wellcome Library.

11. Sappol, *Traffic in Dead Bodies*, details this "male fraternity of dissectors" and its
    carnivalesque actions, 80–88. He notes that there were dangers in the education,
    both moral and medical, in the form of disease and infection. He notes that
    "medical student life was marked by bantering, stag humor, and practical
    jokery—and often enough a flirtation with cannibalism and necrophilia." (84).
    For the record, an important work by John Knox, *The Anatomist's Instructor and
    Museum Companion: being practical directions for the formation and subsequent
    management of anatomical museums* (Edinburgh: Adam and Charles Black,
    1836), instructs the medical profession on how to organize a museum. Clearly
    the intended visitor is more the medical student than the general public; and
    the medical student learns by being involved in its care and keeping. This is the
    same John Knox who purchased corpses from Burke and Hare in the famous
    Edinburgh body-snatching case.

12. This in fact became the primary focus of anatomical exhibitions later in the cen-
    tury when they became associated with the Chambers of Horrors of the Wax
    Museum. Sappol, *Traffic in Dead Bodies*, devotes an instructive chapter in his
    book to the legacy of these museums, which outlived their pedagogical function
    and reverted—or adapted—to the voyeuristic "imperative." See also Leslie Fiedler,
    *Freaks: Myths and Images of the Secret Self* (New York: Simon and Schuster,
    1978), Robert Bogdan, *Freak Show: Presenting Human Oddities for Amusement
    and Profit* (Chicago: University of Chicago Press, 1988), Rosemarie Garland
    Thomson, ed., *Freakery: Cultural Spectacles of the Extraordinary Body* (New York:
    New York University Press, 1996), and Martin Howard, *Victorian Grotesque: An
    Illustrated Excursion into Medical Curiosities, Freaks and Abnormalities, Principally
    of the Victorian Age*, (London: Jupiter Books, 1977) on the widespread display of
    abnormality as "freaks" of nature.

13. The history of early minstrelsy has been written about with enthusiasm almost
    from its inception. T. Allston Brown published what amounts to a (surprisingly
    accurate) documentary history in the *New York Clipper* in an 1876 series, revised
    and expanded in 1912. An abundance of newspaper articles can be found in
    files and scrapbooks in the New York Public Library and the Harvard Theatre
    Collection, among other archives; by their existence and content it appears that
    minstrelsy had a strongly loyal and long-lived fan base, which was keenly inter-
    ested in the originals of the genre and its change over time. For later narrative
    histories, see Carl Wittke, *Tambo and Bones: A History of the American Minstrel
    Stage* (Durham: Duke University Press, 1930), Harry Reynolds, *Minstrel
    Memories: The Story of Burnt Cork Minstrelsy in Great Britain from 1836 to 1927*
    (London: A. Rivers, 1928), Edward Leroy Rice, *Monarchs of Minstrelsy, from
    "Daddy" Rice to Date.* (New York: Kenny Pub. Co. [c. 1911]), and especially
    Hans Nathan, *Dan Emmett and the Rise of Early Negro Minstrelsy* (Norman, OK:
    University of Oklahoma Press, 1962/77) and Robert Toll, *Blacking Up: The
    Minstrel Show in Nineteenth-Century America* (New York: Oxford University
    Press, 1974). The general statements that follow are based on this material, as
    well as books by Lott, *Love and Theft*, William J. Mahar, *Behind the Burnt Cork
    Mask: Early Blackface Minstrelsy and Antebellum American Popular Culture*

(Urbana: University of Illinois Press, 1999), Dale Cockrell, *Demons of Disorder: Early Blackface Minstrels and their World* (New York: Cambridge University Press, 1997), and W. T. Lhamon, *Raising Cain: Blackface Performance from Jim Crow to Hip Hop* (Cambridge: Harvard University Press, 1998), and *Jump Jim Crow: Lost Plays, Lyrics, and Street Prose of the First Atlantic Popular Culture* (Cambridge: Harvard University Press, 2003).

14. For an example of the reference to the early "glut" of minstrels, see *John Bull*, October 24, 1846: "So many things of this kind have been brought forward lately, by Henry Russell, the Hutchinson Family, the Ethiopean Serenaders, and we do not know how many others, that they are getting quite stale; and any further attempt of the sort must have some wholly new features in order to become attractive." Blackface as a theatrical convention was still in use on American and British television in the 1960s. From personal experience, I know that service clubs in North America still used the form as a feature of fund-raising events in the 1980s.

15. *Manchester Guardian*, October 18, 1848, p. 5, col. 4.

16. Lyrics for Lucy Long abound in early minstrel publications. Samples and discussion can be found in Mahar, 307-11, and in Lott, 160-61. The lyrics printed here are from sheet music found in the British Library.

17. Eric Lott's *Love and Theft* examines the complex psychology and politics of that first, working-class audience; Dale Cockrell's *Demons of Disorder* and William Mahar's *Behind the Burnt Cork Mask* examine its roots in folk and popular tradition, and its transition into a commercial form; W. T. Lhamon's *Raising Cain* explores the genre's long-term legacy, and *Jump Jim Crow* the legacy in Southern folk ritual. A range of periodical literature also exists in what has been a rich field of research over the past fifteen years. For reference to Harlequin and minstrelsy, see George F. Rehin, "Harlequin Jim Crow: Continuity and Convergence in Blackface Clowning," *Journal of Popular Culture* 9 (1975): 682-701. For a more wide-ranging discussion of Atlantic culture, see Joseph R. Roach, *Cities of the Dead: Circum-Atlantic Performances* (New York: Columbia University Press, 1996).

18. See *The Libertine*, June 15, 1842, p. 14, col. 2,3 in the archive of the American Antiquarian Society. This image and description are discussed in Cockrell, *Demons of Disorder*, 8-11.

19. For discussions of the effect of a commodity or consumer culture—the "show business"—on folk and popular performance, see Chandra Mukerji and Michael Schudson, eds., "Introduction," *Rethinking Popular Culture: Contemporary Perspectives in Cultural Studies* (Berkeley: University of California Press, 1991), 38-39, discussing Adorno, Michael Schudson, *Advertising: The Uneasy Persuasion: Its Dubious Impact on America Society* (New York: Basic Books, 1984), especially his discussion of "Capitalist Realism," and Jackson Lears, *Fables of Abundance: A Cultural History of Advertising in America* (New York:

Basic Books, 1994). The word "class" is troublesome; its use here should not be misinterpreted as easily defined, monolithic, homogeneous, or discrete. Individuals are "members" of a range of cultures and subcultures, some of which may be defined through class. See with respect to mid-nineteenth-century Anglo-American society: Hugh Cunningham, *Leisure in the Industrial Revolution, c. 1780–c. 1880* (London: Croom Helm, 1980), which outlines three popular cultures expressing hedonism, methodism, and radicalism, 37–41; Bluford Adams, *E Pluribus Barnum: The Great Showman and the Making of U.S. Popular Culture* (Minneapolis: University of Minnesota Press, 1997), which follows Barnum's tactics for appealing to and manipulating a cross-class culture of "respectability"; and Karen Haltunnen, *Confidence Men and Painted Women: A Study of Middle-class Culture in America* (New Haven: Yale University Press, 1982), which explores with elegance the phenomenon of the middle classes as a culture "in social motion" (29). These arguments inform this study, as does Douglas A. Lorimer, *Colour, Class and the Victorians* (Leicester: Holmes and Meier, 1978).

20. Cockrell, *Demons of Disorder*, uses the story of George Washington Dixon extensively in his discussion. Every study of early minstrelsy discusses T. D. Rice, but Lhamon, *Raising Cain*, mines the document most completely.

21. *Morning Post*, June 21, 1848, from a souvenir silk in the Dance Collection, New York Public Library, dated by internal evidence to 1848; also quoted in the *Stirling Journal and Advertiser*, August 31, 1849, p. 4, col. 4.

22. *Morning Post*, June 21, 1848, p. 4, col. 4.

23. *The Manchester Examiner*, October 17, 1848, p. 4, col. 5.

24. See Stephen Johnson, "Testimonials in Silk: Juba and the Legitimization of American Blackface Minstrelsy in Britain," in *Culture of Emulation: The Role of Testimonials in the American Marketplace*, eds., Marlis Schweitzer and Marina Moskowitz (New York: Palgrave Macmillan, forthcoming).

25. *Manchester Guardian*, October 18, 1848, p. 5, col. 4.

26. *Era*, August 27, 1848, p. 11, col. 1. See also *Manchester Guardian*, October 18, 1848, for the following:

> With a most bewitching bonnet and veil, a *very* pink dress, beflounced to the waist, lace-fringed trousers of the most spotless purity, and red leather boots,—the ensemble completed by the green parasol and white cambric pocket handkerchief,—Master Juba certainly looked the black demoiselle of the first ton to the greatest advantage. The playing and singing by the Serenaders of a version of the well-known negro ditty, furnished the music to Juba's performance, which was after this fashion:—Promenading in a circle to the left for a few bars, till again facing the audience, he then commenced a series of steps, which altogether baffle description, from their number, oddity, and the rapidity with which they were executed. The highland fling, the sailor's hornpipe, and other European dances, seemed to have been laid under contribution, and intermixed with a

number of steps which we may call "Juba's own," for surely their like was never before seen for grotesque agility, not altogether unmixed with grace. The promenade was then repeated; then more dancing; and so on, to the end of the song.

27. These admonitions are from a later appearance in Manchester, noticed in the *Era*, August 4, 1850, p. 11: "[Juba is] jumping very fast at the Colosseum, but too fast is worse than too slow, and we advise [Juba] to be wise in time. It is easier to jump down than to jump up"; *Era*, August 11, 1850, p. 12: "Juba has jumped away—by the way of an earnest yet friendly caution, let us hope that he will not throw himself away. Be wise in time is a wholesome motto." See also the *Huddersfield Chronicle and West Yorkshire Advertiser*, November 30, 1850, p. 5, col. 1: "The performances of Boz's Juba have created quite a sensation in the gallery, who greeted his marvellous feats of dancing with thunders of applause and a standing *encore*. In all the rougher and less refined departments of his art, Juba is a perfect master." This review damns by faint praise, a far cry from the rapturous reviews of 1848-1849.

From *The Puppet-Show*, August 12, 1848, in a Harvard Theatre Collection folder devoted to Vauxhall Gardens:

> Juba's talent consists in walking round the stage with an air of satisfaction and with his toes turned in; in jumping backwards in a less graceful manner than we should have conceived possible; and in shaking his thighs like a man afflicted with palsy. He makes a terrible clatter with his feet, not owing so much to activity on his part as to stupidity on the part of his boot-maker, who has furnished him with a pair of clumsy Wellingtons sufficiently large for the feet and legs of all the Ethiopians in London: besides this, he sometimes moves about the stage on his knees, as if he was praying to be endowed with intelligence, and had unlimited credit with his tailor. As a last resource, he falls back on the floor.

28. T. Allston Brown, from "Early History of Negro Minstrelsy—Its Rise and Progress in the United States," an occasional series published in the *New York Clipper*, February 24, 1912.

29. "Exceptional normal" is used by Edoardo Grendi, quoted in Giovanni Levi, "On Microhistory," in *New Perspectives on Historical Writing*, ed. Peter Burke (Cambridge: Polity Press, 1991), 93-113, 109. Other related terms include: "an opaque document," in Robert Darnton, *The Great Cat Massacre: and Other Episodes in French Cultural Life* (New York: Vintage, 1985), 5; a "dissonance," in Carlo Ginzburg, "Microhistory: Two or Three Things That I Know About It," *Critical Inquiry* 20, no. 1 (Autumn 1993): 10-35; and a "contradiction of normative systems," in Levi, "On Microhistory," 107.

30. Most writers of early minstrelsy include a discussion about Juba; most of these are based on the essential article by Marian Hannah Winter, "Juba and American Minstrelsy," in *Dance Index* 6, no. 2, (February 1947): 28-47, in *Inside the Minstrel Mask: Readings in Nineteenth-Century Blackface Minstrelsy*, Annemarie

Bean, James V. Hatch, and Brooks McNamara, eds. (Hanover, NH: Wesleyan University Press, 1996). See also *Inside the Minstrel Mask*, but this is based on a very few documents. Many more are now available for study. See www.utm.utoronto.ca /~w3minstr and http://link. library.utoronto.ca/minstrels

31. As one example, he specifies not only the exact date of death for the performer G. W. Pell, who also figures in this chapter, but also the county, parish, and church cemetery, as if his readers might wish to visit the site. This information was corroborated by—and allowed for the location of—the death certificate. *New York Clipper*, March 30, 1912.

32. Note as examples: *Sheffield and Rotherham Independent*, October 28, 1848, p. 4, col. 6:" Juba is a perfect phenomenon, a genuine Son of the Southern clime, who will introduce the NATIONAL SONGS and DANCES of his country; accompanied by Briggs, on the native Instrument, the Banjo." *Manchester Guardian*, October 18, 1848, p. 5, col. 4: "His other performances were called the 'marriage festival' and 'plantation dances,' in which, in male costume, he illustrated the dances of his own simple people on festive occasions." *Theatrical Journal*, July 11, 1850, p. 222: "We understand, he is a genuine grit negro, from the far-west, and not one of those domestic manufactured piebald abortions of Ethiopianism." *Theatrical Journal*, July 25, 1850, p. 339: "It is laughable betimes to witness the abortive attempts of those collier or whitewashed personations of the Ethiopian. They are just as much in character as a pig is in a drawing-room. Juba's executions are both graceful and accomplished."

33. Marjorie B. Garber, *Vested Interests: Cross Dressing & Cultural Anxiety* (New York: Harper Perennial, 1993), 302, considers the possibility that the "drag" of Little Richard provided his sexual attraction with a "cover," distracting the audience away from race prejudice. See also the image of Juba dancing in Vauxhall Gardens; the audience is comprised entirely of women.

34. Roland Barthes, *Camera Lucida: Reflections on Photography*, trans. Richard Howard (New York: Hill and Wang, 1981), 13, 15.

FOUR

# The "Disabled Imagination" and the Masculine Metaphor in the Works of Leonard Kriegel

HAYLEY MITCHELL HAUGEN

> To experience we have to imagine; imagination is con-
> sciousness struggling to gain sovereignty over its experi-
> ence.
>
> —Arthur W. Frank, *The Wounded Storyteller*

> How odd that we are at once tethered to the truth of our
> bodies and yet, at the same time, utterly free to sculpt
> ourselves.
>
> —Lauren Slater, *Lying*

WRITING *INTOXICATED BY MY ILLNESS* during the last fourteen months of his life while dying from metastatic prostate cancer, Anatole Broyard laments the fact that most narratives about illness and disability focus only on the waking life of the patient and have "little to offer about the imaginative life of the sick"[1]; they do not tell much "about [the patient's] daydreams or fantasies, about how illness transfigures you."[2] Privileging the imagination, Broyard takes issue with Susan Sontag's popular and influential work, *Illness as Metaphor*. Focusing, he says, more on the "conceptualization of illness than [on] the daily experience of it," Sontag is "too hard on metaphors" in her push for a truthful regarding of illness.[3] "While she is concerned only with negative metaphors," Broyard writes, "there are positive metaphors of illness, too, a kind of literary aspirin. In fact, metaphors may be as necessary to illness as they are to literature, as comforting to the patient as his own bathrobe and slippers."[4] Broyard believes in what he calls "the therapeutic value of style," and that "every seriously ill person needs to develop a style for his illness."[5] "Adopting a style for your illness," Broyard writes, "is another way of meeting it on your own grounds, of making it a mere character in your narrative."[6]

It is not surprising that American essayist Leonard Kriegel would find Broyard's work appealing. In fact, Kriegel frequently recalls Broyard in his own essays, and like Broyard, he has had a profound relationship with his own imagination since his polio-related paralysis at age eleven. His autobiographical works not only reflect heavily on the various imaginative views of himself during childhood, but also rely, as Broyard's do, on metaphor as a key component of their style. Just as Kriegel creates a style for his work, he also fabricates a style for his illness.

In Kriegel's first book, *The Long Walk Home*, a memoir published in 1964, the boy, Lennie Kriegel, relies heavily on his own imagination as well as escapist, fantasy-inducing pursuits such as reading and going to movies to get himself through harrowing medical treatments and humiliating public experiences during his treatment and recovery from polio. Lennie was just one of thousands of children to contract the polio virus, or *poliomyelitis*, during the summertime polio epidemics that swept across the United States in the 1940s and early 1950s. Also known as *infantile paralysis*, the acute, infectious disease often caused permanent paralysis in one or more limbs of its victims, as it does for Lennie, who loses the use of his legs to the disease. After this loss, Lennie privately yearns for opportunities to be heroic and beloved by all. Or he simply retreats into his imagination out of hatred of himself and others, fashioning himself in his mind as a pitcher, a boxer, a lover, and more, as he struggles through late childhood and adolescence in search of a new, authentic self.

Kriegel stylizes this theme of imaginative retreat through his use of masculine images and metaphors that have a twofold effect on the narrative and contribute to the sociopolitical nature of his work. Self-fabricated as the hero of his own quest, the boy, Lennie, embraces the masculine imagery of his vivid imagination to gain an immediate sense of power over his sterile medical surroundings. Kriegel, the adult author, however, emphasizes masculine imagery throughout his memoir in an effort to set his work firmly within a tradition of masculine American autobiography, a move that helps counteract the dominant American view of the disabled man—and by extension, the disabled male author—as emasculated.

As Kriegel depicts in *The Long Walk Home*, Lennie relies heavily on his vivid, masculine imagination during his first hospital stay to alleviate feelings of guilt over his disease, fight physical pain, relieve boredom, and to wield as a weapon against "enemy" doctors and nurses. Upon Lennie's waking in the hospital, the doctor, in the true patriarchal spirit of medicine at the time, informs Lennie and his mother that the virus had, Kriegel writes, "ended its frontal attack upon my body. . . . It had stopped its march before it reached the upper part of the stomach."[7] From the start, then, Lennie is encouraged to view the polio virus as an enemy of war, something capable of attacking and marching, and, in his case, retreating before it could do more harm. In his essay "The Body of Imagination," Kriegel says, "the image I chose [for the virus] was taken from the wartime propaganda of comic books and my virus looked like a sinister 'Jap,' America's yellow, bucktoothed, eyeglasses-wearing enemy."[8] Embracing the war imagery his doctor has suggested to him, and influenced by media images of World War II, Lennie hears his doctor barking orders to others "like an army sergeant" (*Home* 19). And he prepares himself mentally for a painful transfer from a stretcher to a bed by imagining himself at war:

> I thought of what I had read about war and suffering and closed my eyes to smell the rain-freshened earth of Normandy, my mind repeating that sound, Normandy, Normandy, Normandy, Normandy. . . . I drove tooth into tooth with that cheap Hollywood consciousness of the victim, a prisoner of the Nazi Gestapo. Then the pain laced from the small of my back to my legs, ankles, feet, toes, to my shoulders, chest, neck, head, until my teeth-grinding courage was shattered by the howl of the shorn Samson in my bones. (Home 19)

In this scene, Lennie attempts bravery by calling up the masculine imagery of war. Though he senses that some of these images stem from Hollywood's cheap fabrication of the courageous hero-victim, he has faith that embracing this kind of masculinity will get him through his ordeal. In this instance, however, Lennie senses an important American belief about disability: His illness is his Delilah; it has the power to emasculate.

The emasculating potential of illness is an important lesson for Lennie to learn early on, as American culture enforces the idea of the disabled as powerless. In his essay "Fighting Polio Like a Man," Daniel J. Wilson explores male polio survivors' response to mid-twentieth-century masculinity. Wilson explains that the polio epidemics of the 1940s and 1950s occurred at a time when many believed that American manhood was in crisis.[9] "Cold war-era cultural critics worried that American men had lost their strength, vitality, and autonomy in becoming victims of a smothering, overpowering, suspiciously collectivist mass society," Wilson writes.[10] With their masculinity already being questioned by American society, disabled men and boys at the time were at greater risk for stigmatization. Wilson quotes Robert Murphy's study of the effects of paralytic illness: "Paralytic disability constitutes emasculation of a more direct and total nature. For the male, weakening and atrophy of the body threaten all the cultural values of masculinity: strength, activeness, speed, virility, stamina, and fortitude."[11]

In an effort to fight the emasculating potential of his illness, Lennie continues to retreat into the masculine scenarios played out by his imagination after he is transferred to the Reconstruction Home in West Haverstraw, New York. During the long days on the ward, he conjures up baseball players smashing homers at Ebbets Field, and he recalls himself performing physically active pursuits. He remembers his first two-wheel bicycle, for example, and the man who used to chase him through the gardens near his home. He recalls a boy in tears whose nose he bloodied after being called "Christ killer" (*Home* 36). In each of these images, Lennie recalls himself or others excelling in tasks requiring physical strength. He is unwilling to let go of his image of himself as the strong, physically active boy he once was before his fight with polio.

Lennie's feelings of nostalgia are complicated, however, by his conflicting feelings about his approaching manhood. In the weeks before his bar mitzvah, for example, he is troubled by the thought of leaving the hospital for the day and "facing the world [he] had known before the virus" (*Home* 110). He does not rejoice in this important celebration of his manhood, and he dreads the pity others will feel for him. As if to confirm his fears, when Lennie arrives at the synagogue, there is no wheelchair access available, and the stone steps leading up to the portal have no banister that would allow him to climb them on his own. Rather than entering through the front door, he must use a side entrance where his father and a taxi driver have to lift him over a couple of short steps to a landing (*Home* 113). From the door he must walk twenty feet to the podium set up for him in front of the rows of seats. He is unable to walk the distance without stopping to rest, and when he reaches the front, Kriegel recounts, "my father and a member of the congregation picked me up and carried me up the four marble steps onto the podium" (*Home* 114). Lennie is literally carried into manhood.

## FROM FANTASY TO REALISM

Lennie's new manhood is soon marked by another beginning, his being discharged from the hospital and returning home as effectively "cured." Whereas a traditional restitution narrative would describe this event as a time of triumph, Kriegel marks this period in his life as another one of adversity. His recovery and rehabilitation prepare him to move around in the world successfully, for the most part, but they do not prepare him to *live* in it. They do not make him a man. Sensing this fact, Lennie does not look forward to leaving the comfort and safety of the hospital and returning to his old Bronx neighborhood, where he is especially concerned about falling in public. In rehab, he tells his friend,

> We all fall. It's like we all eat and sleep and go to physio. Here, it's natural. But that's not what I'm scared of... what about when you're lying on the ground [outside the Home and in society] and you look up and there's some bastard shaking his head. It's pity. That's what it is for him. And then you have to ask him to help you. What about that?" (*Home* 50)

For four years after returning home, Lennie avoids this possible scenario by spending most of his time indoors, retreating again into fantasy, where he can construct himself as a powerful, able-bodied hero: "Reality shredded into a million scattered pieces as my mind performed its ritual dances," Kriegel writes, "—ball player, union leader, soldier, lover, fighter, killer, politician, doctor, lawyer, Indian chief. Nothing could interfere. Nothing" (*Home* 148). Uncertain about his own manhood, he continues to embrace the masculine heroes of sports or famous men making the evening newspapers, in an effort to move "away from the reality the mirror told me was mine," Kriegel confirms. "Reading, listening to the radio, anything that allowed me to detach myself from the crippled adolescent I really was. I became an even more avid baseball fan, for now that I couldn't play I needed even more the stimulus of evaporating into myth. I was Pete Reiser or Pee Wee Reese, rarely Lennie Kriegel" (*Home* 129).

When Lennie becomes fearful of his future, his fantasy world is a comfort to him. Like his favorite Hollywood actors, he can slip easily into any role he wishes to play. When he wonders, "How do you become a man without legs? Can you touch a woman without legs?" (*Home* 130), he reminds himself of this easy availability of fantasy: "Importance, dignity, these belong to you too," Lennie tells himself. "Keep them. But never forget, when it becomes too tough, you can be Pete Reiser or Eugene Debs. Never forget that" (*Home* 130). In his essay "Homage to Barney Ross" in *Falling into Life*, Kriegel reiterates the importance of fantasy in his life. "Fantasy proved a gift both of and for the disease-ridden imagination," he writes. "I owe my virus that much. For it was the disease-ridden imagination that recognized that before the day came that I could claim myself, I would have to claim all my imaginary selves."[12] That Lennie finds these imaginary selves through the masculine role models of baseball players and other sports figures is significant for Kriegel's narrative. First, Lennie is trying to recapture a sense of the boy he was before his illness. Before he was stricken by polio, it is clear in the narrative that Lennie took pride in his strong body and that sports were important to him. Kriegel recalls, "I was big for my age, strong, a rather good athlete, which is always the holed ace in a young boy's quest for leadership" (*Home* 6).

Lennie, to be sure, will always be interested in sports; athletics are ingrained in his psyche. It is also interesting to note, however, that sports metaphors are commonly found in polio narratives. In his essay "Covenants of Work and Grace: Themes of Recovery and Redemption in Polio Narratives," Wilson studies the narratives of about fifty people with polio (including Kriegel), represented in twenty-five book-length autobiographies and biographies published between 1947 and 1989, and twenty-eight shorter pieces published between 1936 and 1991.[13] In part, Wilson finds that therapists, doctors, and nurses all "responded to the disease and to the rigors of rehabilitation by relying on familiar images and metaphors. The medical professionals sought to inspire their patients by appealing to the widespread notion that hard work inevitably brought rewards. For others imbued with competitive instincts, a sporting challenge served to motivate."[14] This covenant of hard work, Wilson contends, enabled patients to "regain some sense of power, some sense of self, in a life shattered by disease."[15]

Kriegel taps into the images inherent in the covenant of hard work, as Wilson describes it, especially in viewing the virus, at times, as a sporting challenge. It is possible that these images may be ingrained in him through his experience at the hands of the patriarchal practitioners that made use of these same images for motivational purposes. America's expectations for men and boys during the 1940s fueled these images in an era when, as Kriegel writes in his essay "Taking It," a man was "expected to face adversity with courage, endurance, determination, and stoicism" (*Life* 55). Polio, especially, he feels, "was a disease battled by being tough, aggressive, and decisive. And by assuming that all limitation could be overcome, beaten, conquered. In short, triumph over polio's effects lay in 'being a man.' One was expected to 'beat' polio by outmuscling the disease" (*Life* 56). In his research, Wilson discovers that Kriegel is not the only male writer to present polio as a disease meant to be tackled like a man, "rejecting dependence and passivity in favor of actively resisting the limitations imposed both by a crippled body and by an unaccommodating society."[16] Although he does not specifically discuss these images at length in the works by the authors he studies, Wilson finds, in fact, that similar myths of the warrior and the athlete helped numerous youths through their recoveries. Rather than succumb to the emasculating effects of their illness, the men in Wilson's study embraced "the cultural values of masculinity—strength, aggressiveness, toughness, activity, stamina, and fortitude—[that] were allies in the struggle to recover muscle function and to achieve something approaching a normal life."[17]

While this tough, resilient thinking was a part of the lexicon of American medicine at the time, Wilson fails to note that Lennie's reading about ball players or fantasizing about being a sports hero is also, clearly, very much his own way of expressing his masculinity and the kind of manhood he desires. In addition, Kriegel's work is essentially different from the other polio narratives Wilson describes because most of Lennie's masculine triumphs occur only in his imagination. In admitting this, Kriegel complicates the usual "triumph over adversity" story, offering a counternarrative not only to American culture's view of the ill and disabled, but to polio survivors' views of themselves.

Lennie's fantasies, then, are only triumphant in that they offer him a means of escape. As the "'real world' grew more difficult and less appealing," Kriegel writes elsewhere, "I bombarded myself with images of muscular prowess" (*Life* 43). In one such fantasy, Lennie imagines himself as a heavyweight championship boxer while getting his legs massaged during therapy:

> It became one of my most enjoyable fantasies. As Mr. Courant massaged my dead knees and calves, I would rehearse the fight, slowly coming out of my corner, hands knotted into two huge fists, protecting my face, stalking my opponent. The thrill of the warrior's approach with the knowledge that I was already the victor, cleansed and purified by the effort of my dream, my opponent's face a penitential mask for all those who had ever hurt me....(*Home* 145)

In fantasies such as this one, Lennie privileges the violence and physicality of masculine brute force. He fantasized about fighting, Kriegel writes in *The Long Walk Home*, because he worshiped power (44). And in his prizefighting fantasies, he sought something different than in his fantasies of other sports:

> It wasn't the resurrection of movement I craved, nor was it the almost unbearably sweet memory of the tingling sensation in my wrists as bat connected with ball. I depended upon my fantasies about fighting for something deeper, a sense of myself as still possessing the very power whose absence threatened to destroy me even as I dreamed, spurred on by my weakness. (47)

Whether dreaming about the athletic prowess of baseball players or the masculine power of boxers, for four years Lennie avoids life outside his Bronx apartment in favor of the life he lives within his vivid imagination. Kriegel admits, "if life was frequently no more than a fantasy, it was, at times at least, a rich one" (*Home* 147). And, if only temporarily, Lennie's rich fantasy life fuels his image of himself as a man. At the movies, especially, he can retreat into an "afternoon dream of manhood," where nothing can hurt him (*Home* 142). While he watches Gunga Din, Jesse James, or a charge at Iwo Jima, all of Lennie's feelings of "impotence, confusion, withdrawal, terror, and shame died during those rich hours in the dark, [his] body straight and strong and sure now, [his] mind the king of its own custom" (*Home* 142). In fantasy, Lennie triumphs, but he is acutely aware that his imaginative victories are fleeting, as when he leaves the movie theater—wearing his leg braces and using his crutches—to find the light "exposing the reality that was I as I walked back up Bainbridge Avenue, my head still full of dreams, but the alley of salvation closing around me as the eyes that belonged to others pierced time to tell me that I had to wait for the next week to live" (*Home* 142). When Lennie approaches his seventeenth birthday, he abruptly discovers that an internal life of fantasy can serve him only so far, that despite his masculine fantasies, he eventually always has to return to the real world where he feels, inevitably, that he is less a man. He still has to face society, and society sees him as a cripple. In growing older, Lennie says that "simply by the power of a greater mobility I would not admit to myself I didn't want, to get around more and more in that world below my window, I found it more and more difficult to maintain the myth" (*Home* 149).

The myths of his childhood are, in fact, shattered when Lennie succumbs to a case of boils: "And that was where my new man was conceived," Kriegel quips, "—in bed with boils" (*Home* 149). After his release from the rehabilitation center, Lennie experiences boils as a regular nuisance as a result of walking with his leg braces and crutches. The apparatuses irritate his skin, causing painful abscesses that become horribly inflamed with infection. Usually, he looks upon them as an opportunity to stay indoors and daydream, escaping the "eyes that burned through me in the streets" (*Home* 149). On this occasion, however, his boils are especially painful. As he looks upon the stickball game his brother and his friends are playing down in the street below his window, he attempts to slip into the "familiar, comfortable, reassuring" daydream of becoming whichever one of them he wanted to be (*Home* 149). But as he watches, the boils ache, "contracting with meticulous regularity" (*Home* 150). Unlike in the past, Lennie cannot ignore the pain of the boils, a pain so insistent it interferes with the masculine myths he has embraced so dearly for the past four years:

> the boils just throbbed, like a neon sign flashing on and off, on and off, on and off. And then the myths dropped away forever, to die permanently in a sudden burst of anguish and despair. Because *I was a cripple.* Not a ball player, not a hero, not a lover, not even an adolescent, but a cripple. Nothing but a cripple. And now each contraction of pain said to me, "You are a cripple, a cripple, a cripple." That was all—so simple, so

brutal, a truth, the kind of truth I had never before permitted to invade my consciousness, a total candor that came with all the shock impact of an idea that was to embed itself permanently within the boundaries of my existence. *I was a cripple.* (*Home* 150)

With this realization, Lennie's masculine fantasies fall away; crying, he turns from the window to mourn them.

Whether inspired by boils or baseball, whatever tears Lennie sheds over the loss of his childhood myths are quickly replaced by anger, as he comes to embrace the reality of his life. He promises to take control over his own body and "show them all," by molding the "fat of my body into muscle, until my body could do whatever my mind ordered it to do" (*Home* 152). In this brief but life-altering moment, the hate boils up in Lennie; it "knotted in [his] stomach and gave way to a dry, hard rage" (*Home* 152). This anger, however, is cathartic. In recounting the boils experience again in his essay "A Few Kind Words for Anger," Kriegel explains, "Anger taught me that I could still make demands upon mind and body, that to be a cripple did not mean that one was relieved of the obligation to be a man. If anything, to be a cripple meant that the need to be a man was stronger and even more decisive."[18]

Now feeling a need to assert some control over society's construction of him as a cripple, Lennie bids farewell to the imaginative realms of childhood and channels his anger into a new obsession with exercise—an effort to strengthen his arms and mold his body into a literal masculine form. Wilson argues that Kriegel's mission to change himself through physical therapy and exercise suggests that he "accepted the covenant that hard work promised victory over the virus."[19] In Wilson's study, however, hard work and receiving God's grace are closely aligned in ways we do not see in Kriegel's narrative. Wilson contends that a covenant of grace is present in the rehabilitative efforts of nearly all the polio survivors in the narratives he studies. They strive to "achieve some level of understanding, some sense of acceptance and resignation, or some faith in God's ultimate purpose as a means of coming to terms with their remaining disability"[20]; they "find grace, acceptance, and redemption with what the virus has left them."[21] This sense of grace, of accepting God's wishes, Wilson adds, often coincides with newly found or newly strengthened religious faith, so that "the experience of polio only confirmed [patients'] belief in God."[22] Without this experience of grace, Wilson writes, without this redemption, "these healing stories could not have ended in their characteristic triumph over polio."[23] Kriegel, however, as noted previously, provides a counternarrative to these other polio narratives, with their decidedly conversion-like undertones. When recalling his purpose for writing his illness narrative, Kriegel admits that he wanted to "write a book free of the sentimentality and cant and papier-mâché religiosity usually found in such books" (*Life* 87). Illness narratives or fictional works overflowing with religious sentimentality, he writes, "work to disguise disease and disability and encourage the ill and disabled to simply 'trust in God's goodness and man's charity' rather than their own goodness or their own abilities" ("Imagination" 26).

As a nonbeliever, Kriegel writes elsewhere, he feels that "the cripple's presence merely testified to a calculus of accident. One could accept the implication of such mathematics, since one's acceptance was beside the point. Both believers and nonbelievers were powerless to change the way things were" (*Life* 177). In *The Long Walk Home*, the teenaged Lennie clearly rejects God, and he is not open to receiving his grace. Kriegel concedes, however, that "something in me was desperately looking for salvation when I was sixteen and lay in bed with boils."[24] He finds this redemption through the power he wields over his own body. Exercise, Kriegel writes, "was the first step toward selfhood," and "in the arms was my salvation" (*Home* 154). Wilson concedes that "grace might also come in more secular guises," and that Kriegel's obsession with exercise serves as a "*kind* of redemption" for him (emphasis mine).[25] Later, however, Wilson maintains that "grace and redemption have proven elusive for Kriegel," a statement that I believe belittles Kriegel's feelings about the importance of exercise during this time in his life.[26]

Kriegel also admits in the narrative, however, that he realistically understands that his obsession with exercise is perhaps another form of fantasy:

> But it was fantasy that had nothing to do with an imaginative life. I had to protect the growing self within me, to nurture the awakening power of my body, to break through all the old possibilities my imagination had offered into the promise of real selfhood. To be! That was it. I had to be. (*Home* 154)

In this mind-set, Lennie retreats from the world around him and into an "embryo of selfhood" nurtured through exercise. He does pushups in his room until he collapses in pools of sweat, considering each painful lifting of his body as a "victory" over everything he hates (*Home* 155). And this hate carries him through an hour's workout before breakfast, two hours of "brutal exercise" after his hour of home-schooling, and, later in the day, twenty-block walks through the neighborhood, wearing his braces and crutches, "the muscles in [his] shoulders so swollen with fatigue and pain that each step was a burning screw twisted deeper into [his] flesh" (*Home* 155). After dinner, Lennie's grueling routine continues, as he walks to the city park for an additional two- to three-hour workout on the monkey bars (*Home* 156).

Lennie's desire to better his body is productive in the sense that the strength he gains from his efforts offers him both greater mobility and a healthier psyche in the end. On the other hand, Lennie's family expresses concern over his manic exercise, but he refuses to listen to their pleas that he take things more slowly. In fact, he turns away from his family and friends altogether in favor of his pursuit of bodily strength. And as he grows stronger and proud of losing weight, he becomes increasingly self-confident and self-reliant. For instance, he loses his old fear of doctors and nurses. Once the enemy, they now seem "ridiculous" to him as he works gracefully with the weights and parallel bars during his weekly rehabilitation (*Home* 158). Most importantly, he proves, in their presence, that he no longer needs their—or anybody's—assistance, for "by this time," Kriegel writes, "I had learned how to balance all my weight on one arm while doubled over and boost myself with the other arm on a single crutch—an important victory, for it freed me of asking for help when I fell" (*Home* 158).

After losing thirty pounds and gaining immense strength in his upper body during his summer of exercise, Lennie believes "that the world now envied my grace and courage, just as I had once believed that the world had fathered my fatness, my helplessness, my terror" (*Home* 160). For the first time, Lennie feels like a "man among men, notwithstanding knees that were strapped to steel" (*Home* 160). Kriegel, however, notes his own naïveté in this passage, hinting to readers that Lennie's victory is not complete, despite his new feelings of masculinity: "It didn't occur to me then, that the world did not care, that it was as indifferent to me and to my triumph as it was to everyone else" (*Home* 160).

In a significant scene, it becomes clear that Lennie's temporary manic existence has not alleviated his concern over how others view him. Despite perfecting his upper body, he still feels the stigma and shame of his disability. At midsummer, Lennie is puffed with pride over his bodily transformation, a change he sees as a "healthy, childish, brutal game called 'getting even'" (*Home* 161), and he looks forward to a trip to a mountain lake retreat with his family. Feeling that his newfound manhood is "invincible" (*Home* 162), Lennie plans a water ritual through which he can cleanse away the last remnants of adolescence and emerge a man. Recalling looking out over the water of the lake, Kriegel writes, "It was here that I would do it. My sex, my manhood, my power, my destiny, the end of the adolescence I had never had—it lay on the surface of the lake, as cold and green and wet and waiting as the water itself" (*Home* 162). The next day, Lennie rows out to the middle of the lake with his brother. He takes off his pants, unstraps his leg braces, asks his brother to row twenty feet ahead of him, and slips cautiously into the water (*Home* 162).

As Lennie swims, he feels that "neither time nor memory" can hurt him (*Home* 163). Relaxing, he floats on his back a few moments before he swims "savagely," triumphantly to the other shore (*Home* 163). Kriegel describes his feelings of invincibility in the water:

> The water, the sun, the dock at the other end of the lake, the obliteration of time, the manhood I was reaching for—these were all waiting for me. And I was never going to die. I knew that as I cut through that water, because I was somehow bigger and better and taller and smarter and higher and lower than anything or anyone that had come before me. Like God, I was. (*Home* 164)

Lennie's great swim is a powerful and moving scene in the narrative. Readers rejoice in his physical triumph and believe, as he does, that he will be reborn out of water into the manhood he has been seeking. The scene is made more poignant, however, by the fact that Lennie's victory is short-lived. His arms, made strong enough through exercise to propel him across the lake, have not, in the end, propelled him toward redemption. He is not the god, after all, that he imagined himself to be. As Lennie pulls himself up on the dock, he rejoices in his victory while putting his shoes and braces back on. Suddenly, however, he feels self-conscious, worrying that someone may see his braces, his atrophied legs, from shore. In this brief moment of self-consciousness, Lennie makes an important discovery: "I had won over the lake," Kriegel writes, "but I had lost the real victory in my fear of being seen. My body remained an anachronism, a cripple's body. And no matter how many pushups I had done, no matter how many lakes I would swim, I remained ashamed of revealing that body to others" (*Home* 164).

In acknowledging the shame he feels in what otherwise would be a moment of triumph, Kriegel also acknowledges that, for him, rehabilitation of the body does not lead to triumph over his disability. Even at age seventeen, Lennie is acutely aware of the degree to which his disability and his sense of self are socially constructed. Not until he comes to terms with the social stigma of his disorder will he find the "authentic" self he has been seeking. His efforts are hindered, however, because despite all he has learned about the pitfalls of embracing a masculine fantasy of himself, masculine posturing has been ingrained in him through American culture. This same summer, Lennie feels the negative effects of this cultural influence on his first date, when he falls in front of his date and feels emasculated in her presence:

> Barbara picked up the crutches. She had a certain sure dignity of touch that gagged me for the moment, holding the crutches as if they were not wooden crutches but rather spears, clean and agile and shafted in their

ability to pierce flesh. I knew little enough about the terror of the phallus then but it was with me for sure. This was my potency, my strength; like Samson's hair, this was the feeder of my manhood. I pushed up straight, using one crutch hand to boost myself, then grabbing the other crutch from Barbara's hand. (*Home* 168)

As Barbara enters her hotel, Lennie hates her for having tried to soothe him, for trying to make him feel less embarrassed, and for brandishing against him the tools through which he displays his masculine physical strength as weapons. Given the 1940s script of masculinity that Lennie is following, it is not surprising that he feels threatened in this scene. He is not yet emotionally capable of accepting Barbara's gesture of comfort.

Exhausted from the long walk and feeling "weak and flabby," Lennie turns to head back to his own hotel, determined to refuse rides from passing cars. The length of his journey is, of course, suggestive, as Lennie finds himself on yet another long walk home. In a rage of humiliation, he cries as he walks into the night, feeling he has lost an important battle. Kriegel recalls that he was crying because

Barbara's softness had turned to stone in my hands, crying because the fever in the blood was now no more than the desire not to be humiliated any further, crying because I had come so close to the greatest and most necessary of all the incestuous loves, the love of the self, only to have it wrenched from my grasp. (*Home* 169)

By the time he reaches his hotel, Lennie is at the peak of his rage, vowing revenge on everything. He spends the next day in a whirl of self-pity, feeling that the "world was rancid with the smell of my disease" (*Home* 170). Ultimately, though, Lennie finds that his defeat with Barbara is a minor one. In time, his emotional wounds heal and Lennie ultimately reaches a point in his life where falling in front of a woman has a much less dramatic outcome.

*The Long Walk Home* ends on a positive note, with Lennie feeling that he has paid his debt to polio and discovered his authentic self. There is a sense that his physical, emotional, and social battle with the virus is over. As Wilson correctly notes, however, Kriegel's

subsequent essays over a quarter of a century recount his continuing struggle to make sense of his crippling, to reshape a usable past out of the chaos of pain and limitation. . . . [He gives readers] some insight into the continuing struggle that is the lasting legacy of polio. Kriegel's accounts of this forty-year struggle to create a self starkly reveal the difficulty of sustaining affirmation or triumph over a lifetime marked by pain, disability, and limitation.[27]

A year and a half after the publication of *The Long Walk Home,* Kriegel first learns that the effects of polio will be lasting when he breaks his wrist in a fall. The incident makes him realize that the virus would not only "stimulate and irritate" him for the rest of his life, but also become the obsession of his future writing. "The virus had created me," he writes. "The virus had been transformed into the mote in the writer's eye. In taking my legs it had given me a way of looking at the world and at myself. Nothing I would ever write would be free of its legacy" (*Life* 87).

Kriegel understands, then, that his illness and disability pervade his whole life, and it is through embracing illness and disability that he finds—and writes—his authentic self. He is primarily an autobiographical writer, and his illness story informs, if not dictates, the bulk of his lifewriting. Indeed, Kriegel's body of work is unique in that it gives us a writer's perspective on his illness through the decades; Wilson notes that only two other writers in his study write more than one account of their polio experience. In continuing to write about disability as a lifetime challenge, Kriegel offers a more realistic model that contends that living with chronic illness and disability is a constant battle. With this contention, he provides a counternarrative to the medical model of illness and disability that considers the struggles of the ill and disabled as effectively over once their bodies are rehabilitated and they no longer need immediate medical care.

What is especially interesting about Kriegel's body of work from a literary perspective, though, is that he not only provides counternarrative to society's dominan discourse on disability, he provides counternarrative to his own work. In his continuing search for authenticity, he is not afraid to reevaluate the ideas in his own writing. The conclusion of Lennie's narrative, for instance, reads: "At the cost of legs, I had won a self. How much cheaper a price could I have expected to pay?" (*Home* 213). However, in his essay "On Manhood, Disease, and the Authentic Self," written fifteen years after the publication of *The Long Walk Home,* Kriegel admits to feeling much differently about the ending of the memoir:

> I can think of no sentence as singularly untruthful as that last. I would give a great deal to be able to take it back today. For I know now how truly expensive such victories are, how fragmentary, how terribly short-lived, how ludicrous to call the price "cheap" and how essentially demeaning to the legitimate and painful demands I had made upon myself....The price is never cheap. And that authentic self is never quite won.[28]

The lesson that living with chronic illness or permanent disability is a lifelong battle is a valuable lesson for the ill and disabled who have sought solace in illness narratives that tell them to surrender themselves to American medicine, or to God, or to simply grin and bear it while their physical and social trials continue. Kriegel's narratives, then, come closer to representing a broader range of experiences and emotions that a larger population of both disabled and ablebodied persons can relate to than traditional restitution and conversion narratives manage to do.

## FROM ILLNESS, THE WRITER'S VOICE

Nearly thirty years after the publication of *The Long Walk Home*, Kriegel's life comes full circle, as he once again embraces the vivid imagination he rejected as a teenager in favor of sculpting his body. Now, however, he recognizes in his writing that it is his body and the polio virus in particular that have given him a writer's voice. "For it was that virus," Kriegel writes, "which taught me how to see and what to look for. And it was that virus which forced me to recognize that in writing about who I was and how I lived, I was still speaking for that eleven-year-old boy, the *who* I should have been and the *how* I might have lived" (*Life* 85). Indeed, for over forty years Kriegel has made his reputation as a writer by mining what he calls the "imagination housed in the damaged body" ("Imagination" 29). He knows that "as a writer [he has had] to conceive of the life not lived [a life without polio] in order to understand the life lived" (*Life* 86).

Kriegel explains that "cripples" living consciously as "cripples" are constantly obsessed with their bodies, an obsession that affects their imagination as well as their use of language. In his essay "The Body of Imagination," Kriegel notes other ill and disabled authors for whom the body has become imagination's focus. Illness or disability has made or "remade" them as writers (26). For these artists, Kriegel argues, "the body lurks like some giant termite gnawing at the imaginative life we knew before illness had control not only of our physical existence, but also of our sentences" (25), but he also discovers that "to enter what Susan Sontag called the 'more onerous citizenship' of illness is to discover that language can defend the broken body" (29). Kriegel not only feels this way about his own work; he recognizes a similar role in the imaginations of other contemporary disabled writers:

> The multiple sclerosis that forces [Nancy Mairs] into a wheelchair also gives her strategies for survival and strategies for imagination. Writing about the life that illness makes her live, she must speak of the life she has been prevented from living. This is the price the crippled writer pays.

> One is always imagining what might have been if....We are different
> from normal writers because for us the imagination is housed in the dam-
> aged body. ("Imagination" 29)

Arthur W. Frank likewise contends that tellers of illness stories are different from other writers in the way that their illnesses not only interrupt
their lives but also disrupt their memories. "The memory that is disrupted
is a coherent sense of life's sequences," Frank writes; "the present is not
what the past was supposed to lead to and whatever future will follow this
present is contingent."[30] Frank's ideas here pertain to Kriegel in the sense
that he views his writing as a way to seek revenge on the past that interrupted his present. Always haunted by what might have been, Kriegel has
continued to examine the life unlived in his work:

> Desire is always linked to memory, and the literature of bodily affliction
> turns on the moment before illness imprisoned the writer in her dead
> limbs or cancerous growths or the exhaustion of the effort he must make
> to get into a car. It is not much in the way of compensation to note that
> only words can resurrect the time before one had to combat the anguish
> of the broken body. The reader may find inspiration in those words. But
> all that the writer finds is loss revisited and the sound of imagination—
> screaming. ("Imagination" 30)

Today, as Kriegel examines the life lived against the unlived life, his imagination not only continues to scream, it continues to embrace the masculine imagery and metaphors that served him so well as a child recovering
from the effects of polio, and as an adult writing about those effects in *The
Long Walk Home.*

As Wilson notes in "Fighting Polio Like a Man," Kriegel, like many
polio survivors, has experienced post-polio syndrome, now decades after
his initial rehabilitation. The symptoms of post-polio syndrome include
"new muscle weakness, increased fatigue, increased muscle pain, decreased
endurance, and the loss of hard won function."[31] For men, Wilson adds,
post-polio syndrome "poses new challenges to their masculinity. The hard
won victories of rehabilitation are slipping away, and the metaphors of
battle and competition that sustained their youthful struggles against the
disease have lost their power to inspire and motivate."[32] Ultimately, Wilson
finds that the "masculine ethos that had spurred [the men's and boys']
recovery could not always be sustained over a lifetime of living with a disability; rather, these men have "had to alter their relationship with their
disability and their sense of manhood as they aged."[33]

Kriegel has written about his own struggle with post-polio syndrome in
his essay collection *Falling into Life.* Wilson recounts Kriegel's struggle

briefly in his own essay, focusing on Kriegel's return to using a wheelchair full-time for mobility. Kriegel's return to the wheelchair is symbolic of letting go of the masculine defiance that fueled his insistence on walking with braces and crutches through most of his adult years. As evidence that his definition of masculinity has changed as he has aged, Wilson notes Kriegel's surprising finding that returning to the wheelchair was not the "'spiritual death' he had feared."[34] Wilson adds, "after forty years of crutch-walking, forty years of struggle, defiance, and resistance, it was time to say 'no more,' and to recognize that he had put up a good fight but that the time for that particular fight had passed."[35] What Wilson fails to notice, however, is that although Kriegel's views on masculinity may have changed in regard to his wheelchair use, he still embraces mid-twentieth-century ideas and images of masculinity in his current work. As the title of his most recent collection of essays, *Flying Solo: Reimagining Manhood, Courage, and Loss*, suggests, Kriegel has continued to grapple with the meaning of these images—the meaning of manhood—throughout his life. And just as masculine themes have remained prevalent in his work, masculine metaphors have not lost their power to inspire and motivate him—only whereas they once inspired Kriegel's will to triumph over the body, they now inspire his writing.

## CONCLUSION

Still writing, publishing, and publicly reading his work today in his early seventies, Kriegel maintains these obsessions. In his essay "Superman's Shoulders: On the Healing Power of Illusion," for instance, Kriegel is inspired by the death of actor Christopher Reeve to reflect on Reeve's quintessential role as the man of steel in Hollywood's series of *Superman* films. Kriegel admits to delighting in Reeve's portrayal of the comic book superhero who once tantalized his imagination as a boy. Kriegel was drawn to Superman as a boy of seven, but after he contracted the polio virus, the superhero came to mean even more to him as he developed an "unabashed passion" for Superman's shoulders, in much the same way that he came to love his own strong shoulders that he relied upon to carry him on his crutches: "In the secret alleys of imagination, their strength was as mythic as Superman's. A cripple learns to love what he needs—a boy with dead legs needs nothing more than strong shoulders."[36]

   With aging, however, Kriegel's strong shoulders begin to rebel against him with the pains of arthritis and bursitis, and the death of Christopher Reeve reminds him of his own mortality. But Superman, Kriegel argues, essentially died eight years earlier, when Reeve's spinal cord was crushed in a horse-riding accident: "The fall that made him a cripple made the world's most powerful body an object of pity, transforming the Man of Steel into a creature so frail that it was dependent on machines to breathe and electric chairs to move" ("Superman" 5). When Reeve dies, however, his death affects Kriegel as no other had in recent memory, not because his beloved Superman was lost forever, but because he had been inspired by Reeve's refusal to accept his fate and by his believing in "the illusion of invincibility":

> he lived his final years trying to come to terms with what every cripple must sooner or later come to terms with—to recognize that determination, courage, and will are simply not enough, that no matter how tough one may be one must still confront the rage of all the humiliations fate imposes on the body, and that even a body of steel can be forced to acknowledge the passive daring that every cripple must claim if he wishes to be independent. ("Superman" 7)

Reeve's "passive daring" was embodied in his belief and public insistence that he would walk again. Kriegel admired Reeve's "insistence that bodily resurrection was a real possibility," and even though Kriegel himself has been crippled since age eleven, he believed Reeve's claim that he would walk again ("Superman" 8). He salutes Reeve's rejection of those in the medical community who encouraged him to give up the illusion of recovery and to embrace rehabilitation efforts instead, and he views Reeve as a new kind of Superman, one who "assumes defiance for everyone forced to live with a broken body" ("Superman" 10). Part of Reeve's defiance that Kriegel honors was his refusal to "glory in being crippled for the sake of what is now called 'the handicapped community'" ("Superman" 10). Reeve would not become a spokesperson for this community, and "his insistence that he would walk again was mocked" by disability rights activists who "viewed such desires as treason" ("Superman" 13). The handicapped community hoped Superman could help "make being crippled acceptable," but it was not acceptable to Reeve: "That he refused to surrender his dream of triumphing over what broke him was his heroism" ("Superman" 13). Kriegel honors Reeve for being "brave enough to resist the world's demand that he behave realistically" and for holding tight to the "healing power of illusion" that Kriegel himself responded to as a crippled boy, fantasizing about running, and that he responds to now, "still dreaming of hitting a baseball and running through grass and what sand feels like between the toes," understanding, as Reeve did, that it is "more courageous to live with illusion than without it" (14–15).

Holding onto his 1940s childhood illusions of masculinity may date Kriegel too much for some of today's readers. His obsession with manhood and masculine imagery remains fascinating nonetheless, especially in light of the different ways that Kriegel returns to these obsessions over and over as he ages and gains new insights into the events of his past and the cultural moment of postwar masculinity, now long gone. The enduring quality of Kriegel's work lies not in the endurance of these topics and images, however, but in how, in Kriegel's hands, these very specific, personal events of his life remind all readers what it is to be human, what it is to suffer human pain.

## NOTES

1. Anatole Broyard, *Intoxicated by My Illness* (New York: Fawcett Columbine, 1992), 16.

2. Broyard, *Intoxicated*, 14.

3. Broyard, *Intoxicated*, 18.

4. Broyard, *Intoxicated*, 18.

5. Broyard, *Intoxicated*, 25.

6. Broyard, *Intoxicated*, 62.

7. Leonard Kriegel, *The Long Walk Home* (New York: Appleton-Century, 1964), 14-15. Hereafter cited in the text as *Home*.

8. Leonard Kriegel, "The Body of Imagination," *Nation*, November 9, 1998, 25. Hereafter cited in the text as "Imagination."

9. Daniel J. Wilson, "Fighting Polio Like a Man," in *Gendering Disability*, ed. Bonnie G. Smith and Beth Hutchison (New Brunswick: Rutgers University Press, 2004), 120.

10. Ibid., 120.

11. Ibid., 121.

12. Leonard Kriegel, *Falling into Life* (San Francisco: North Point Press, 1991), 54.

13. Daniel J. Wilson, "Covenants of Work and Grace: Themes of Recovery and Redemption in Polio Narratives." *Literature and Medicine* 13, no. 1: (1994): 25.

14. Wilson, "Covenants," 31.

15. Wilson, "Covenants," 31.

16. Wilson, "Fighting Polio," 119.

17. Ibid., 121.

18. Leonard Kriegel, *Flying Solo: Reimagining Manhood, Courage, and Loss,* Boston: Beacon Press, 1998, 54.

19. Wilson, "Covenants," 28.

20. Ibid., 24.

21. Ibid., 25.

22. Ibid., 33.

23. Ibid., 24.

24. Leonard Kriegel, "In Bed with Boils: Literary Realism as Salvation's Mentor," *Ohio Review* 51 (1993): 67.

25. Wilson, "Covenants," 34, 35.

26. Ibid., 37.

27. Ibid., 38.

28. Leonard Kriegel, "On Manhood, Disease, and the Authentic Self," *Nation*, August 11, 1979, 120-21.

29. Kriegel notes, in order, Nancy Mairs, Andre Dubus, Stanley Elkin, Anatole Broyard, Paul Monette, and Harold Brodkey. Kriegel provides a helpful list of suggested readings by these and other authors at the end of his essay, from which I began much of my own study of illness narratives.

30. Arthur W. Frank, *The Wounded Storyteller* (Chicago: University of Chicago Press, 1995), 60.

31. Wilson, "Fighting Polio," 128.

32. Ibid., 128.

33. Ibid., 127.

34. Ibid., 129.

35. Ibid., 129.

36. Leonard Kriegel, "Superman's Shoulders: On the Healing Power of Illusion," 3. *Southwest Review* 91, no. 2: (2006): 258-67.

FIVE

# Of Genes, Mutations, and Desires in Franz Kafka's *The Metamorphosis* and Moacyr Scliar's *The Centaur in the Garden*

CATALINA FLORINA FLORESCU

> You are more and more authentic the more you like
> someone you dreamed of being.
> —Pedro Almodóvar, *All about My Mother*

ONE OF THE BOLD QUESTIONS addressed in Susan Sontag's book *Illness as Metaphor* is whether or not a society could catch a (fatal) disease. While Sontag is particularly focused on a society in which citizens are diagnosed with cancer, my chapter takes a look at individuals whose bodies lose their human carnality and become animals, as in Franz Kafka's 1915 *The Metamorphosis*, or return to their human shape after an animal phase, as in Moacyr Scliar's 1983 *The Centaur in the Garden*, and how this metamorphic process affects a society.

The main argument that connects these novels is based on the notion of the dys-appearing body. As defined by Drew Leder in his book *The Absent Body*, in such a state "[t]he body *appears* as thematic focus, but precisely as in a *dys* state—*dys* is from the Greek prefix signifying "bad," "hard," or "ill," and is found in English words such as "dysfunctional.'"[1] Leder argues further that a body could "dys-appear" (as opposed to "disappear,"

---

To my father, in his memory, To Mircea, my son, my passion

for example, the body at partial rest, during sleep) when one is diagnosed with a terminal illness as well as when one finds oneself in severe hunger, thirst, and/or weakness. How could we better define this phenomenon? What are its implications? How does one exist in a body that is dys-appearing? These are some preliminary questions that frame my chapter.

It is worth noting that just as there occurs a physical dys-appearance of the body in severe pain, there might also be a social dys-appearance. In the second type of malfunctioning, "[t]he split is effected by the incorporated gaze of the Other. [. . .] A radical split is introduced between the body I live out and my object-body, now defined and delimited by a foreign gaze."[2] Those in abominable pain are confronted not only with their acceptance of having a body different than it used to be, but also being unjustly marginalized, isolated in hospitals, asylums, etc. What Leder may imply is that the gaze of the other thematizes the body. To take the issue of thematization a step further, we could suggest that illness itself thematizes a body. We do not (or rarely) see our own body because we are sculpted into it, and consequently barely notice its evolution (or should I say involution?). But how could we exist outside of our body and still somehow be aware of it? Does only the encounter with an illness remind us that we have a body?

Furthermore, whether in good or poor health, how do we perceive and transform our body into bodily narratives? "In an age of volatile extremes," such as ours, "the body has become another realm of fantasy."[3] We are assembled and assembling machines, made of congruous as well as incongruous parts. Memory, and along with it the sum of our fulfilled and unfulfilled needs, plays a substantial yet tricky role in the assembling of life. We remember events distortedly because time melts away the fringes and, more often than not, the contents of our narratives. The closer we attempt to move toward the epicenter of our lives, the more difficult it becomes for us to untangle its labyrinthine structure. In his book *Phenomenology of Perception*, Maurice Merleau-Ponty writes: "My body is the fabric into which all objects are woven, and it is, at least in relation to the perceived world, the general instrument of my 'comprehension.'"[4] But what happens when the fabric of the body breaks? As we shall see, the literary works chosen for interpretation in this chapter focus on two examples of a "body-broken"; they also form a pertinent example by adding another component to suffering and dys-appearance, i.e., mutation. In these works by Kafka and Scliar, pain is visualized either as a metaphorical exhumation of the animal lurking beneath the well-camouflaged site of the human or the human reemerging out of the animal cocoon.

To understand this transformation, or breakage, it is worth asking this question: How do we define pain? According to Susan Greenfield, "[w]e know pain is expressed as other associations: pricking, stabbing, burning, chilling. [...] We [also] know that the more people anticipate pain, the more they perceive it as painful; and I would suggest that that is because there is a build-up of neuron connections."[5] We may say pain is one constant in our fleshy ontology. When in pain, the body—or the affected bodily area—is thoroughly sensed by us, giving us the impression we are locked in our body. This phenomenon is known as "coenesthesia," or "[t]he general sense of bodily existence. [However, when in pain,] we are no longer dispersed out *there* in the world, but suddenly congeal right *here*."[6] Particularly related to the works discussed here, regardless of how these authors decide to approach the theme of pain *as* bodily mutation and imprisonment in "here," the animal (centaur) and insect (bug) involved in these transformations are terrifying, disturbing, yet eerily fascinating. The outcome of combining and grafting human tissues onto their animal counterpart brings into focus the hybridity of the project, along with its ethical questions (addressed later in this chapter).

For the moment, suffice it to say that the theme of mutation has ancient origins. In Greek mythology, a chimera (and chimera-like creatures) was considered a hybrid animal, having the body of a goat, the head of a lion, and the tail of a serpent. As Suzanne Anker and Dorothy Nelkin write, "[c]himeras once populated the literature, mythology, and art of ancient Greece. They were dangerous, formidable, and powerful beasts, representing fantastic yet uncivilized and chaotic forces in nature that confronted mankind."[7] However, to ground the discussion of this theme only in literature would be to limit its vast implications. Instead, in analyzing the experience of pain of Kafka and Scliar's characters, we may learn not only how to be more sympathetic toward the pain of the other, but also acknowledge that "[t]hrough sound, through the various refrains, we invent, repeat, and catch from non-humans, we receive news of the cosmic energies to which we humans are always in close, *molecular* proximity."[8]

We may have actually crossed the line of "molecular proximity" and redirected ourselves toward a borderline physical identity. Transgenic experiments, for instance, have been conducted since the end of World War II. "Bioengineers have created sheep-goat chimeras, known colloquially as 'geeps,' and transgenic pigs that produce low-cholesterol meat."[9] Ironically, while our carnality has been deeply influenced and/or altered by scientific experiments that keep it at a debatable ethical intersection between what is human and what is animal, when in pain, we have not yet learned how to howl at the moon. In other words, to regulate our pain, we depend almost exclusively on medical prescriptions; yet, as I show in this chapter, there is a social component of pain that cannot be treated with drugs.

## GREGOR SAMSA HAD A DREAM

We come into this world on a cradle of dreams, and we continue to dream throughout our lives. We keep our eyelids shut for a while, hoping to reach beyond the limitedness of our given spatial-temporality. We feel a thrill at the mind's fracturing and relocating itself toward places saturated with our creating and populating of the world. A few dream to destroy and harm ourselves and others, but even fewer awake to find their human, vibrant carnality transformed mockingly into the disturbing shape of a gross insect. This is the experience Kafka's main character in *The Metamorphosis* undergoes: "As Gregor Samsa awoke one morning from an uneasy dream, he found himself transformed in his bed into a gigantic insect. [...] What has happened to me? he thought. It was no dream."[10]

Shocked by this transformation, he desperately clings to his mind, the last vestige of a once used-to-be-*exclusively*-human site: "And at all costs he [Samsa] must not lose consciousness now, precisely now."[11] Does the human, recording yet self-effacing mind, reel backward, hopelessly trying to unearth the meaning of the human condition? What type of dys-appearance does Samsa experience? Kafka does not offer much about the origin of Samsa's transformation. Nonetheless, his character's experience is profoundly shocking; one day he wakes up differently, not as a human being, but in the shape of a bug. What Kafka may imply is that his character suddenly realizes he cannot use his body any longer, and thus feels it as a destitute yet burdensome-to-wear *shell*. As Merleau-Ponty suggests, in such unfortunate cases,

> [i]f the world is dislocated, this is because one's own body has ceased to be a knowing body, and has ceased to draw to get all objects in its own grip; and this debasement of the body into an organism must itself be attributed to the collapse of time, which no longer rises toward a future but falls back on itself.[12]

Furthermore, as he sadly acknowledges, Samsa suffers a double shock, if not an insurmountable disappointment. On the one hand, he is confronted with a new carnality whose nature not only alarms him but also of which he does not know much, let alone accept. On the other hand, he must face the disgust and shame of his family when they see him:

> Slight attacks of breathlessness afflicted him and his eyes were starting a little out of his head as he watched his unsuspecting sister sweeping together with a broom not only the remains of what he had eaten but even the things he had not touched, as if these were now of no use to anyone.[13]

If Samsa suffers from an enigmatic mental and corporeal collapse, and taking into account his family's cold and unsupportive reaction, could we go further by suggesting that anomalies function similarly to a contagious disease? Or why do we believe that the body without anomalies would remain unchanged? The body is in continuous motion and, therefore, transformation. As Bryan Turner points out,

> [b]ecause embodiment has in fact many dimensions, one can talk about having a body in which the body has the characteristics of a thing, being a body in which we are subjectively engaged with our body as a project, and doing a body in the sense of producing a body through time.[14]

The body as a project has an unfinished quality, a suspension of disbelief vis-à-vis its mortality. It is reminiscent of the Deleuzian and Guattarian "BwO," body-without-organs. In *Medicine as Culture: Illness, Disease and the Body in Western Societies*, Deborah Lupton notes,

> [t]he body-without-organs is much more than the material or anatomical body (this is, the body-*without*-organs). It is the body self, the "self-inside-the-body," a phenomenon that is cognitive, subconscious and emotional as well as experienced through the flesh.[15]

However, when we live with a body whose inside begins to collapse and deteriorate as Samsa's does, the body becomes compartmentalized and *with* organs. In other words, though we could easily engage in endless discussion about the unfinished quality of the body, in reality nothing unsettles and troubles us more as when our body falls (seriously) ill. Those are the moments when we wish our body were a "finished" project, remaining the same, unaltered.

> "In German," Hans-Georg Gadamer writes, "a doctor will begin by asking, 'Na, wo fehlt's denn?,' or 'What is the matter with you then?,' literally, 'What are you lacking?' [...] Is it not an extraordinary thing that the lack of something, although we do not precisely know what it is that is lacking, can reveal the miraculous existence of health? It is only now, in its absence, that I notice what was previously there."[16]

Etymologically, "absence" is a derivative of *esse* ("to be") with the significant irony that it adds an "ab" ("away") to *esse*. In other words, something is added that steals from being. Just as we do not have one body but several embodiments, comparatively we experience several absences (some productive, others destructive) from our being-in-us and being-in-the-world. In this light, when Teresa de Lauretis writes "[e]xperience is never *im*-mediately accessible,"[17] what she may imply is that a person constitutes him-/herself as subject if and only if his/her subjectivity becomes temporarily blocked by objects upon which to contemplate and events by which to be intrigued. Otherwise, without this suspension from one's experience, there would be an unproductive and disturbing continuum of ego-subject-subjectivity. An experience that is never "im-mediately" accessible may also mean that there is a necessary rupture not only between the subject immersed into seeing and reflecting upon an object, and sometimes upon him-/herself as an object, but also of life consisting of inescapable moments of partial absences.

One classical example of partial absence is experienced during sleep, when our turmoil is put on hold by disseminating the self into dreams. According to Sue E. Cataldi,

> [n]ight [...] envelopes me and infiltrates through all my senses, stifling my recollections and almost destroying my personal identity. [Night] is pure depth without foreground or background, without surfaces and without distance separating from me. This "pure" depth presents itself as a candidate for the "absolute" space.[18]

Unfortunately, whether at night or during the day, Samsa does not experience the space surrounding him as being infinite. On the contrary, he may feel this space and his presence in it as closing more and more with each day passing. Thus, not comfortable with his new condition and without support from his family, Samsa thinks he does not have any option other than to accept his suddenly undesired transformation. As a consequence, he maddens himself: "[h]e began now to crawl to and fro, over everything, walls, furniture, and ceiling, and finally in his despair, when the whole room seemed to be reeling around him, fell down onto the middle of the big table."[19] He repeats this agonizing ritual until deciding to put an end to his already physically and socially dys-appeared body by committing suicide:

> The decision that he *must disappear* was one that he held to even more strongly than his sister, if that were possible. In this state of vacant and peaceful meditation he remained *until the tower clock struck three in the morning.* [...] Then his head sank to the floor of its own accord and from his nostrils came the last faint flincher of his breath.[20]

Samsa suffers from an inexplicable mutation whose etiology baffles everyone. He does not have a human body anymore, but rather bodily sequelae which, having been pressured by physical pain and social alienation, have resulted in his current deteriorated state of being. In 2002, Pat Croskerry—a physician—wrote the article, "Achieving Quality in Clinical Decision Making: Cognitive Strategies and Detection of Bias," where he states that doctors have a tendency to diagnose their patients after just a couple of routine and rather informal dialogue exchanges and minimal check-ups. Croskerry explains this approach by saying that doctors have a template of diseases, just as, comparatively, literati have a template of tropologies, mathematicians a template of numbers, and art historians a template of genres.[21] Because the human body is a highly heuristic site where several discourses overlap, we have the moral obligation to insist that doctors avoid a perhaps too quick, formulaic diagnosis—understanding by this that, in most cases, signs of an ulterior bodily breakage are evident even before our appointments with doctors.

However, Samsa seems to be the medical enigma par excellence, or the "noncase" of medical cases. Could Kafka, then, be arguing that treating an illness implies an unavoidable degree of isolation, a distortion of personality and a mutation of identity? Since we do not know the exact nature of Samsa's transformation, does his situation imply that we could be transformed against our will? One day, could we become Samsa, that is to say, unrecognizable to ourselves and others? If pain validates a passing through life, and if the encounter with pain cannot be minimized, what should be the next step? According to David B. Morris, "[t]he behaviorist begins from the proposition that all pain can be redefined as pain behavior."[22] For a better understanding of pain, he suggests a suturing between physical and mental pain. In doing so,

> We [would] recover a sense of the importance of minds and cultures in the construction of pain, and we [would] begin to proliferate the meanings of pain in order that we do not reduce human suffering to the dimensions of a mere physical problem for which, if we could only find the right pill, there is always a medical solution.[23]

However, for Samsa there is no available drug to alleviate his agony. Perhaps unintentionally, Kafka offers a further step in the concept of dys-appearance. His character commits suicide, thus totally disappearing. In this light, it is relevant to note the differences between the two concepts: While dys-appearance implies a body still somehow alive, disappearance includes death.


## THE CENTAUR

While in Kafka's story Samsa simply, though inexplicably, awakes in the shape of a bug, in Scliar's novel *The Centaur in the Garden* there is a more intricate scenario. By the time we complete the reading, we discover that there is no clearly defined identity for the main character. What this author proposes for himself as a writer—and for us as readers—is to imagine a character whose inner and outer contours, dimensions, and perceptions are never fixed, but mutable and interchangeable. Moreover, he also suggests that when realities are insufficient to understand who we are, we create myths, novels, and the like. As Scliar suggests, we are more than humans; we are centaurs, Sphinxes, or any other mythological creature superimposed imaginatively on our human identity. In this scenario, life seems unfathomable, unreachable, and unpredictable: "We must contrive to understand how, at a stroke, existence projects round itself worlds which hide objectively from me."[24]

When Guedali, the main character, was born, he had an uncertain biological identity, half-human, half-animal. Shocked and disgusted, his mother could barely look at him, let alone nurture him: "Her [Guedali's mother] silence is an accusation to her husband: It is your fault, Leon. You brought me to this place at the ends of the earth, this place where there are no people, only animals."[25] In order to understand the mother's bitter reaction, it is relevant to note that she and her husband were Russian immigrants in Brazil. This raises the question of whether the place of our birth is pure coincidence, something accidental? Or to the contrary, does it engrave within us the social "genes" of our cultural identity? All those who decide to leave their country of birth experience various degrees of nostalgia, metaphorically translated into mutations and emotional mutilations of various kinds.

For Guedali, the problem is yet of an additional nature. Having been born hybrid, he is equally confused and fascinated by his physicality. He finds relaxation, ease, and pleasure in galloping for hours over the vast Brazilian pampas: "This gallop. This gallop in the middle of the night, through open fields, through swamps that reflect a pallid moon, this gallop is to stay in my memory for many years."[26] When he does not gallop, he reads feverishly, searching for an ancestor to his blessed or cursed fate, but his endeavor is futile. He does not find anything or anyone even remotely related to his unusual condition. The more he searches, the more frustrated he becomes. Finally, he embarks on a cruise to Morocco, where the lower part of his body will undergo a dramatic surgery. The surgery proves to be a success, if not a medical marvel; the centaur's marks of his identity are surgically removed and replaced with human equivalents, for example, hooves with human feet. Still, he has to wear trousers and boots to protect areas of his body not yet fully recovered. For this reason, he feels that someday someone will find out the truth: "What if, one day, I had to have an urgent operation? [...] Or if someone spied on us inside the house, with binoculars? (As to that, I had already taken the precaution of buying thick curtains)."[27] What Scliar may be implying is that, despite the sum of our efforts to fit into society, we never know for sure when and/or how to please it. After surgery, and much to his disappointment, Guedali discovers that people who have been born without an anomaly, *but* are poor and disfranchised, are considered freaks too—a category from which he thought he had escaped surgically.

Baffled by an unwelcome reality that he cannot fully anticipate, Guedali does not feel completely fulfilled or protected at home either, an experience he "shares" with Kafka's Samsa. He is deeply confused. Are his surgery and sacrifices validated? Instead of finding soothing answers to his problematic ontological questions, he becomes more and more alarmed and agitated. He hopes that by reviewing his past life, he will find the link missing from his "evolutionary" process, and thus be able to attach it and recover his identity. He discovers the opposite:

> A centaur, with great effort, becomes a man; later, he goes through a crisis and decides to become a centaur again; then he does not really know if he wants to be a centaur again or not; meanwhile, he meets a crazy sphinx who wants to transform him into a lion man! Ridiculous. Mythological delirium.[28]

What he uncovers is that at the foundation of a person—as well as a society—there are dreams, but there are nightmares, too. There are actualized, mature desires, but there are also repressed desires that (could) return as agonizing pains. The mythological delirium is just another way of pointing to the state of confusion that permeates the fabric of our body as well as society.

In the end, does Guedali choose to remain human or centaur? His epiphany reveals his nature. Guedali is not just a combination of animal and human, but a symbiosis of elements, manifested in one: vegetal, mineral, animal, and human—just as we are since these four elements have altered our shapes and personalities. In this context, an emblematic passage that defines Guedali occurs when he encounters Lolah, the Sphinx. He declines to answer her famous ontological question; instead, he releases her in ecstasy by pleasuring her. Above all, Guedali is a man of the senses. Indeed, his inner world is sensual.

However, if we think that sensuality is the tone with which Scliar concludes the novel, we are bitterly mistaken. The last chapter functions as a contra-argument to the narrative developed thus far. Or perhaps it is metafictional—combining and engulfing a story within a story. Consequently, the overall structure vis-à-vis the book is like a vortex, centripetal, a mise en abîme provoked by Scliar with one possible intention: to let us discover the multifold narrative dimensions of a literary work.

Just as our coming in and out of life is a mystery, so is the process of reading and making sense of a book: "One's first memories naturally cannot be described in conventional words. They are visceral, archaic. Larvae in the heart of the fruit, worms, wriggling in the mud. *Remote sensations, vague pains.*"[29] Memories and realities mix together, fictionalizing themselves. Anything could potentially happen, even in a novel. Scliar twists the end of his novel so drastically that, when one closes the book, one is left dumbfounded: Was Guedali a man? A centaur? Or perhaps a cancer patient? In the last chapter, Tita—Guedali's wife—narrates the story from her perspective. Again, as in Kafka's story, the style is ambiguous. Apparently, Guedali's "Morocco story" took place when he had surgery related to cancer, though we are not given details about it. To deal with chronic pain, and most likely the effects of medication, Guedali experiences amnesia by projecting himself as a centaur. As Greenfield points out,

> Pain is absent in dreams, and that is a small assembly state. Similarly, morphine gives you a dream-like euphoria: the way morphine works is via a natural opiate which acts to make the brain cell assemblies less efficient at being corralled up—therefore, people will often say that they feel pain but it no longer "matters," it is no longer significant to them.[30]

Even bodies in severe pain and physical deterioration could (and some actually do) continue to function because they have mastered the language of habit, even though they now perform it with their last physical resources. The well-known chemist Ilia Prigogine spent a good portion of his research focusing on what he called "far-from-equilibrium" systems; for these unstable systems "a fluctuation can become a bifurcation point or a site of a swerve, where the system spontaneously chooses a path that no scientist can predict."[31] Furthermore, "Prigogine contends that, even in its most complex and indeterminate state, a physical system continues to possess a kind of intelligibility."[32] If bodies in severe deterioration could be read as "far-from-equilibrium" systems, then this kind of intelligibility is a consequence of them having been engaged in performing habit.

However, Guedali might have wanted to forget about his illness. "Nociceptive" refers to something that causes pain. Or, according to the *Online Medical Dictionary*, it is "[t]he process of pain transmission, usually relating to a receptive neuron for painful sensations."[33] In taking these definitions into account, Guedali might have deliberately recreated his new identity as a centaur because his experience of cancer had taught him new habits. After all, surviving cancer (or any other terrible misfortune) implies accepting being different, that is to say, changed. In Guedali's words,

> The story [Tita's] is as ingeniously woven as a soap opera. With one single objective: to *convince* me that I never was a centaur. [...] I still see myself as a centaur, but a centaur growing constantly smaller, a miniature centaur, a microcentaur. [...] Maybe it would be better to let him [the centaur] go, to accept this reality they want to impose on me: that I am a human being.[34]

For most of the novel's readers, the ending is what disappoints them: Why would an author want to recreate a totally different story at the end? For many readers, the ending of the book is an anticlimax. For other readers (as I), the ending, with its story turned upside-down, is the beginning of traveling beyond what is in the book. Still, no matter which interpretation prevails, doubtless we can agree that by the end of Scliar's book, our hearts are racing faster, just as fast as Guedali's hooves galloping across the plains, running away from the "normal" people who are finally *just* human. Ironically, the idea of "normality" proposed by Scliar is impoverished; those who have forgotten to be mineral, vegetal, animal, human—and I would add textual—are limited, the "abridged normal." Or, as Pierre Baldi writes in his book, *The Shattered Self: The End of Natural Evolution,*

> [i]n ancient times we thought that we were made of a stuff completely dif-
> ferent from, say, rocks, or that we were very different from other animals
> or plants, and that we occupied a special position in nature. [Today we
> know that] *homo sapiens* is made of atoms, like all other macroscopic
> objects we know.[35]

Can we ever escape our fear of living life as freely as possible? To answer this question, there is one myth that needs to be destroyed, and that is the myth of happiness. We have been told that this life is nothing more than a series of pains cut short by joys. At the end of life, there is the afterlife with its uncountable blessings. Why do we still follow this myth today? Happiness, like our passing through this life, is *not* a myth. *Heureusement*, Guedali chooses (and teaches us) otherwise. According to him, the flesh and blood of our ontology is the sum of what we have desired and dreamed about, achieved and failed. In his particular case, the moment he seizes his chthonic structure, he may begin to be happy and complete:

> I began to think about buying some land, if possible near the place where
> we had our farm [as a child]. [...] What I wanted was contact with the
> earth—an experience that I considered profound, visceral. I wanted to be
> barefoot, I wanted to grow calluses on the soles of my feet, to make them
> even tougher, even more like hooves.[36]

The dys-appearance of Scliar's Guedali, however, reads differently than that of Kafka's Samsa. After years of searching for validation for his mixed and complex identity, Guedali dys-appears in his essence by his own will. In this "place," dreams and nightmares about his identity may return, but he seems to have accepted them.

There is yet one more piece that needs to be added to decipher Guedali's story. This reading relies on Arthur Frank's 2002 memoir, *At the Will of the Body: Reflections on Illness,* which he composed post factum—namely, after he recovered from testicular cancer. He narrates his experience of cancer in reverse, though reminding readers that this strategy is simply a stylistic excursus into his physical past and that his intention is to keep his mind and body in their present embodiment. Frank does not see any possibility for recovery without anchorage in the present, an idea that Guedali also intuits.

Frank, thus, prompts two puzzling ideas. From what we have noticed so far, both pain *and* recovery reside in the present, sometimes making it difficult to differentiate between the two. Frank is visited by uncertainty, too, when he cannot distinguish between what it is to be healthy and what it is to be ill. As he points out,

> [h]ealth and illness are not so different. In the best moments of my illnesses I have been most whole. In the worst moments of my health I am sick. Where should I live? [...] In "health" there can only be fear of illness, and in "illness" there is only discontent at not being healthy. In recovery I seek not health but a word that has no opposite, a word that just is, in itself.[37]

Frank gives here a carnal definition to a more and more forgotten, steeped-in-routine body; until a diagnosis, breakage, or rupture has occurred, we think of the body as just being "out there." However, even this vague idea could be symptomatic that something is wrong with the way in which we conceive of the body. Rather, a diagnosis, breakage, or rupture may allow us to acknowledge that the body traverses a stasis in which there is a delicate balance (if not an interchangeability) between concepts of health and illness, treatment and recovery. Etymologically, *convalescere* is a Latin word meaning "to grow strong." Invariably, growing strong and/or recuperating is done through resting. But resting in cases of illness often implies sleep and medication. As Frank writes, "I have learned that the changes that begin during illness do not end when treatment stops. [...] Those ill persons who recover must recover not only from the disease but also from being a patient."[38] His alternative, or compromise, is to think of (his) cancer as being in remission, where he oscillates between "periods of activity and treatment. [...] People in the remission society notice details more, because illness teaches the value as well as the danger of the everyday."[39] In so thinking, he admits that his body may break yet another time. Therefore, he emphasizes the crucial element that defines our lives, namely the inescapable randomness that sometimes ignores our plans, needs, and desires and challenges us to confront the breakage in our routine.

Undoubtedly, Guedali is not aware of Frank's concept, where recovery from an illness is perceived as remission. Nonetheless, like patients whose intuition is sharpened by the onset of an illness and treatment, Guedali senses that his remission could best be expressed through galloping. He knows that being confined to a hospital bed comes at the loss, even if temporarily, of bodily motility. After his surgery, then, he envisions himself as a centaur who runs free on the Brazialian pampas.

## CONCLUSION

Kafka and Scliar demonstrate allegorically that matter is in continuous motion. There is one way to think of matter as transforming according to its inner structures, and thus not overstepping dangerously the threshold between the human and nonhuman, the normal and abnormal. Yet there is a totally different effect when matter is seen as transforming into something unpredictable and unrecognizable that defies common sense.

Within the range of exuberance and innocence to maturation and annihilation there are uncountable stages of fear derived from the entropic identity of our bodies. In these stories, we have noticed how two characters undergo severe physical and mental transformations. Could we suggest that, at some level, science itself has undergone a dramatic transformation? Has science evolved or involved? As Jennifer Terry points out,

> [n]ow, in the late twentieth century, after revelations about Nazi medicine, after invention of the nuclear bomb and germ warfare, and after the ecological horror wrought by technological developments, many of us have developed a very skeptical view of the doctrine of rationality and its practitioners.[40]

Furthermore, "We are living now in the age of the magical sign of the gene. [...] Scientists promise that if we can figure out the exact function and location of genes within the human body, the human population could be rid of diseases and defects."[41] We can infer that human beings are on the verge of crossing *the boundary* of being human, and are thus advancing toward hybridity. New shapes for our bodies have already been engineered and advertised in mass-media outlets—prosthetic devices, artificial hearts and kidneys, transplants, xenotransplants, cosmetic surgery, drugs. As suggested in *The Metamorphosis* and *The Centaur in the Garden*, and taking into account the technological delirium in which we live, to be *mise en corps* suggests a conglomeration of socially mediated altered and altering building blocks of physicality and technology, which adapt to each other either organically or by force. While these works treat such transformations/mutations allegorically, on the other hand,

> [b]iotechnology applications involve the creation, combination, and construction of animals to contain the genetic traits of several species, including

human being. Similar to a collage, transgenic animals are an aggregation of extant materials. Genes are reassembled and recombined to create more efficient and profitable "super-animals" for food or pharmaceutical production, to develop research models for neurodegenerative diseases, and to expand further the sources of tissue and organs rendered available for human transplantation. [42]

Admittedly, today it is a challenge, if not an impossibility, to maintain an exclusively human identity throughout our lives. Our contours and shapes are more and more blurred. Based on the works discussed here, could we conclude by saying that a person-patient, who gradually loses his/her carnality, eventually becomes a body-without-*objects*? That is to say, person-patients may experience corporeal liminality not only from within as an undesired effect of their illness, be it mental or physical, but also from without as long as they cannot anchor their interest and perception in any object.

As Cataldi remarks, "[i]t is because of the percipient side of our flesh—this sensitive 'other side of our body' and its distancing from the depth of perceptible flesh—that we are 'incomplete,' as a riddle, gaping, open."[43] We did once venture to fail, and then answered correctly the Sphinx's riddle. Does she know how to answer *our* riddle? Perhaps we have been, and still are, dreaming of a body that has never been born; or, once born, does not know its limits and is, thus, eternal. Perhaps this happens precisely because of our recurrent dream of immortality where we have dared to defy our ontological status. As always, after briefly sojourning and disappearing into immortality, that is to say, after having committed mental hubris, we fall and fold back into ourselves, necessarily fabricated by imagination.

## NOTES

1. Drew Leder, *The Absent Body* (Chicago: University of Chicago Press, 1990), 84.

2. Ibid., 96.

3. Suzanne Anker and Dorothy Nelkin, *The Molecular Gaze: Art in the Genetic Age* (Cold Spring Harbor, NY: Cold Spring Harbor Laboratory Press, 2004), 185.

4. Maurice Merleau-Ponty, *Phenomenology of Perception*, trans. Collin Smith (New York: Taylor & Francis, Inc., 2002) 273.

5. Susan Greenfield, "Inner Space," in *Space in Science, Art, and Society*, eds. François Penz, Gregory Radick, and Robert Howell (New York: Cambridge University Press, 2004), 19.

6. Leder, *The Absent Body*, 75.

7. Anker and Nelkin, *The Molecular Gaze*, 107.

8. Jane Bennett, *The Enchantment of Modern Life: Attachments, Crossings, and Ethics* (Princeton: Princeton UP, 2001), 168, emphasis added.

9. Anker and Nelkin, *The Molecular Gaze*, 90.

10. Franz Kafka, *The Metamorphosis*, trans. Willa and Edwin Muir (New York: Schocken Books, 1968), 89.

11. Ibid., 93.

12. Merleau-Ponty, *Phenomenology of Perception*, 329.

13. Kafka, *The Metamorphosis*, 108.

14. Bryan Turner, "Biology, Vulnerability, and Politics," in *Debating Biology: Sociological Reflections on Health, Medicine and Society*, eds. Lynda I.A. Birke and Simion J. Williams (New York: Taylor & Francis, 2003), 281.

15. Deborah Lupton, *Medicine as Culture: Illness, Disease and the Body in Western Societies* (Thousand Oaks: SAGE Publications, 2004), 24.

16. Hans-Georg Gadamer, *The Enigma of Health: The Art of Healing in a Scientific Age*, trans. Jason Geiger and Nick Walker (Stanford: Stanford University Press, 1996), 74.

17. Donna J. Haraway, *Simians, Cyborgs, and Women: The Reinvention of Nature* (New York: Routledge, 1991), 142.

18. Sue E. Cataldi, *Emotion, Depth and Flesh. A Study of Sensitive Space: Reflections upon Merleau-Ponty's Philosophy of Embodiment* (New York: SUNY Press, 1993), 48.

19. Kafka, *The Metamorphosis*, 119.

20. Ibid., 135, emphasis added.

21. Pat Croskerry, "Achieving Quality in Clinical Decision Making: Cognitive Strategies and Detection of Bias," *Academic Emergency Medicine*, 9 (2002). Croskerre identifies several biases: 1. "anchoring bias," where "[c]ombinations of salient features of a presentation often result in pattern recognition of a specific disease"; 2. "confirmation bias," when accumulated "data can be selectively marshaled to support a favored hypothesis"; and 3. "value-induced bias," when "any biasing tendency toward worst-case scenarios increases the likelihood of detection of diagnosis that must not be missed" (1186).

22. David B. Morris, *The Culture of Pain* (Berkeley: University of California Press, 1991), 142.

23. Ibid., 290.

24. Merleau-Ponty, *Phenomenology of Perception*, 343.

25. Moacyr Scliar, *The Centaur in the Garden*, trans. Margaret A. Neves (Madison: University of Wisconsin Press, 2003), 13.

26. Ibid., 65.

27. Ibid., 108-09.

28. Ibid., 175.

29. Ibid., 7.

30. Greenfield, "Inner Space," 19.

31. Jane Bennett, *The Enchantment of Modern Life*, 101.

32. Ibid., 103-04

33. The Cancer WEB Project, *Online Medical Dictionary*, Department of Medical Oncology, University of Newcastle-upon-Tyne, http://cancerweb.ncl.ac.uk/cgi-bin/omd?query= &action=Home, accessed December 16, 1997.

34. Scliar, *The Centaur in the Garden*, 214.

35. Pierre Baldi, *The Shattered Self: The End of Natural Evolution* (Cambridge: MIT Press, 2001), 11.

36. Scliar, *The Centaur in the Garden*, 182-83.

37. Arthur Frank, *At the Will of the Body: Reflections on Illness* (Boston: Houghton Mifflin, 2002), 135.

38. Ibid., 97.

39. Ibid., 138-39

40. Jennifer Terry, "The Seductive Power of Science in the Making of Deviant Subjectivity," *Posthuman Bodies*, eds. Judith Halberstam and Ira Livingston (Bloomington: Indiana UP, 1995), 137.

41. Ibid., 148.

42. Anker and Nelkin, *The Molecular Gaze*, 90.

43. Cataldi, *Emotion, Depth and Flesh*, 66.

SIX

# The Post-biological Body

## Horror, Nostalgia, and the Visible Human Project

NATALIA LIZAMA

THIS CHAPTER WILL EXAMINE THE National Library of Medicine's Visible Human Project (VHP) and Alexander Tsiaras's *BodyVoyage* CD-ROM.[1] Where theorists such as Catherine Waldby and Eugene Thacker have examined the extratextual and political aspects of the VHP, this chapter will consider both the VHP and *BodyVoyage* in relation to the "post-biological" body, arguing that the post-biological ontology within the VHP and in *BodyVoyage* is concomitant with the elicitation of horror and nostalgia. The VHP, first conceived in 1988, sought to digitize the human body by creating a dataset comprised of photographic, CT, and MRI images of a human corpse. In 1994, the first dataset, named the Visible Male (VM), was created from a male body, and a female body underwent the same process in 1995 to form the Visible Female (VF). The resulting Visible Human (VH) datasets can be processed to create computerized volumetric models of the human body that may be used as the basis for anatomical illustrations, simulations, and software programs. One such program, *BodyVoyage*, in CD-ROM form, constitutes one of many anatomically educational products derived from the VH datasets. Focusing exclusively upon the VM dataset, it enables the user to view the VM body in a variety of ways: as planar slices, animated body fragments, or individual organs.

As will be discussed, the VH body, both as dataset and in its *BodyVoyage* incarnation, is a post-biological one; the VH is reincarnated as digital "flesh" after the biological body has disintegrated beyond recognition. The post-biological ontology enacted in the VHP and in *BodyVoyage* carries with it two distinct tropes of horror and nostalgia. The post-biological horror of the VHP is elicited through the geometric segmentation and mutilation of the deceased body that occurs in order to create its digital counterpart. This horror is further evident in the ghoulish immateriality of the VM within *BodyVoyage*, which is, paradoxically, coupled with a "refleshing" of the VM body through the simulation of three-dimensional space. Post-biological nostalgia in the VHP is closely intertwined with horror, and may be identified in the way that, despite the massive technological mediation involved in the creation of the VH, the project nonetheless promotes the VH as a body whose seemingly "natural" anatomical order has not been altered by technological intervention. This "authentic" pretechnological body sought by the project functions as the irretrievable and longed-for lost object of nostalgia. Within *BodyVoyage*, this nostalgia is manifested through the creation of an "authentic" anatomical body that is nonetheless capable of endless resurrection and manipulation. Both these tropes of horror and nostalgia are consequences of the process of creating a post-biological entity and derive from the recoding of human flesh as digital media that occurs in *BodyVoyage*.

## THE VISIBLE HUMAN PROJECT AND BODYVOYAGE: CREATION AND CONCEPTION

In order to understand the significance of the post-biological ontology of the VHs, it is worth considering the complex process involved in the VHs' transformation from corpse to virtual body. This extraordinary process contextualizes the aspects of the project pertaining to post-biological horror and nostalgia. The cadaver used for the VM was taken from a thirty-nine-year-old prisoner on death row, Joseph Paul Jernigan, who donated his body to the state to be used for scientific purposes after his death. While information about Jernigan's life, including details of his arrest, his death, and even his final meal before execution, is widely available, much less is known about the VF. Other than the fact that the body was donated by a "fifty-nine-year-old Maryland housewife" who died of a heart attack, virtually no other details have been released by the National Library of Medicine (NLM). Although this information about the VF has been suppressed, the selection process involved for both the VM and VF is widely known. The bodies of the VHs went through a rigorous screening process and were chosen from several thousand donated bodies. The aim of this selection process was to find an ideal anatomical specimen devoid of such "abnormalities" as infectious disease, cancer, prosthetics, or bone deformation. Furthermore, the chosen specimen had to have a "normal" physique (neither too fat nor too thin) and had to be less than sixty years of age. In addition to these criteria, the choice of potential bodies was restricted by size, given the limited storage capacity of the laboratory and the size of the imaging equipment to be used.

Jernigan was sentenced to execution by lethal injection after being convicted for murder in the state of Texas. The lethal injection consisted of a massive dose of fast-acting barbiturates that effectively killed him by suppressing his heartbeat; the "advantage" of this form of execution was that it left his organs visibly unaltered. While the body was still warm, it was flown to the NLM laboratory in Denver, where it was X-rayed to detect any physical abnormalities, then scanned to create MRI and CT images, which would later comprise part of the VH dataset. The body was then "sectioned," that is, chopped into four parts by slicing it across the chest, across the upper thighs, and just below the knees, and the resulting four pieces were deep frozen in blocks of blue gel to −70° centigrade. Following this, Jernigan's body was cut transversally into 1mm deep slices that corresponded to the MRI and CT images taken prior to freezing; this was done to enable the body to be photographed at 1mm intervals. The VF's body followed a similar procedure, except that her body was sawn into much thinner slices, one-third the size of those used for the VM's body; she is comprised of 5,189 slices in contrast to the VM's 1,878 slices.[2]

In order to enable photographs to be taken at regular intervals, slices were progressively shaved off the VH bodies, such that, by the end of the process, the body had completely disintegrated and was transformed into a mass of body shavings. Digital images of the body interior were created by photographing the remaining aspect of the body that was exposed after shaving off the 1mm slice (in the case of the VM) or the 0.33mm slice (in the case of the VF). Thus, each digital photograph does not represent an individual slice, but rather depicts a view of the remaining solid body after slices have been shaved off. These photographs, combined with the MRI and CT scans taken earlier, comprise the VH dataset. One of the key features of the VH dataset is its capacity for digital malleability; the entire body or its individual organs can be digitally reconstructed, or viewed from multiple planes and at different locations. Thus, while the original digital photographs were taken along the transversal plane, the dataset can be used to depict the body in its sagittal and coronal planes. The data can also be used to create animated simulations of the VHs, including surgical or investigative procedures, and "flythrough" effect animations that travel through the body layer by layer, as if it were gradually dissolving.[3] The VH datasets can be downloaded, free of charge, from the NLM via the Internet, pending the signature of a licensing agreement. They are comprised of thousands of MRI, CT, and photographic images and are subsequently enormous files; the VM dataset is approximately fifteen gigabytes and the VF dataset, because of the smaller size of the body slices, is approximately forty gigabytes.

Since the completion of the VF in 1995, numerous educational books, animations, and CD-ROMs have been created from the VH datasets.[4] At first glance, it might seem that these various media representations derived from the VHP are in fact secondary to the dataset itself, and therefore perhaps not as culturally notable. Yet this is not necessarily the case; the VH dataset, despite its alleged "free" accessibility via the Internet, is in fact far from free or easily accessible.[5] The enormous size of the datasets means that not only do they require a very large hard drive to be able to store the data (necessitating access to sophisticated and often expensive technology), but downloading these images is extremely expensive, and all but impossible unless working through an institutional server.[6] Even with access to, for example, a university server, the amount of traffic generated by downloading the dataset is very costly, and the process requires an uninterrupted download time of several days.[7]

While the images of the dataset itself are, for all intents and purposes, available to a select few, most of the various publications derived from the VHP are far more accessible to and accessed by the general public. For this reason, the ways in which the VH's digital information is remediated and reconstructed in other media reveals further cultural economies working within the VHP. Of the myriad texts derived from the VH dataset, one of the more fascinating and compelling examples of these is Alexander Tsiaras's BodyVoyage, a CD-ROM software program that focuses exclusively on the VM.[8] The resurrection and remediation of the VHs within the virtual realm of BodyVoyage brings into focus the intricate cultural economies underlying the VHP; just as the VH constitutes a digital remediation of the physical body, BodyVoyage functions as a remediated version of the body of the VH dataset. Moreover, while the premise underlying the VHP is ostensibly one of anatomical education, the presentation of the VH body within BodyVoyage incorporates an aesthetic element not overtly evident in the VHP. In doing so, BodyVoyage works against the premise of anatomical education that permeates the VHP; through this, the post-biological body in BodyVoyage is imbued with a heightened sense of the horror and nostalgia found in the VHP overall.

Indeed, BodyVoyage is perhaps one of the least educational and most spectacular of the various by-products of the VHP, privileging the spectacu-

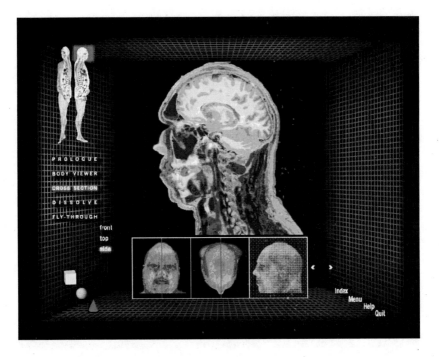

**Figure 6.1.** Cross-section of head from *BodyVoyage* by Alexander Tsiaras. Copyright © 1997 by Alexander Tsiaras. By permission of Grand Central Publishing

larity of the body remediated by technology over any apparent didactic purpose. *BodyVoyage* presents Jernigan's body as a series of disembodied fragments floating ghost-like against a black background, tinted in hyperbright colors. Users of the program can view the body as a whole (Fig. 6.2), or in one of four modules of head, torso, pelvis, or legs (Fig. 6.3). Within each of these modules, there are various commands that can be used to visualize these sections of the body in different ways, such as the "cross-section," where users can view a color cryo-section image from whichever location of the body and plane they choose (Fig. 6.1). There are also "dissolve" animations (depicting animated dissolutions of the body from the top of the head to the soles of the feet) and "fly-through" animations (appearing as if a camera were traveling slowly through a semitransparent body). Perhaps the most compelling images are found in the "Gallery" module, where parts of the body are presented as three-dimensional, semitransparent bodily fragments, brightly colored and turning slowly in multiple directions, framed by a white grid that sits atop a black background (Fig. 6.3). Unlike a typical anatomy text, with its labels and numbers indicating the taxonomy of the interior, *BodyVoyage* gives no explanation of what it

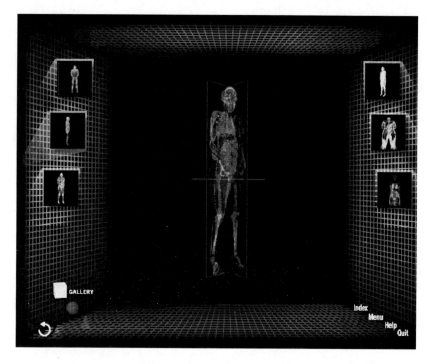

**Figure 6.2.** Gallery module, full body from *BodyVoyage* by Alexander Tsiaras. Copyright © 1997 by Alexander Tsiaras. By permission of Grand Central Publishing

depicts; rather, the images are presented as if affording the viewer a glimpse into a spectacular and otherwise inaccessible vision of wonder.

## THE POST-BIOLOGICAL BODY

The VHs occupy a unique ontological position: while their bodies have long since disintegrated, they continue to "exist" as digital entities within the virtual realm. This transmogrification of the human body into digital information initially seems to be commensurate with Hans Moravec's transmigration scenario.[9] Robotics researcher Moravec envisions a "post-biological" future, wherein human beings gradually evolve to become completely compatible with technology. Within this post-biological future, it will one day be possible to "transmigrate," to download a human being's complete consciousness into a computer, while, presumably, one's remaining body is discarded.[10] This technologically assisted realization of Cartesian dualism will, according to Moravec, endow human beings with

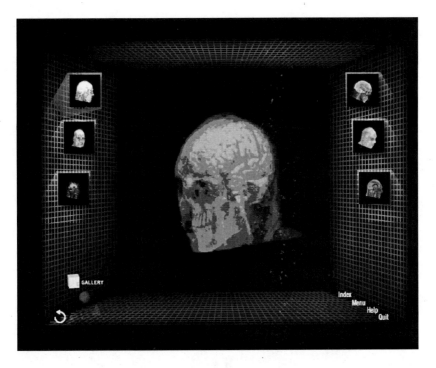

**Figure 6.3.** Gallery module, head, from *BodyVoyage* by Alexander Tsiaras. Copyright © 1997 by Alexander Tsiaras. By permission of Grand Central Publishing

the capacity for post-biological life. Within the VHP, it would seem that, through the transmogrification of humans into data, the transmigration scenario is, in part, fulfilled.

Yet, rather than the minds of Jernigan and the Maryland housewife being transposed into digital information, it is instead their bodies that have been virtualized, while their subjective consciousnesses are no longer embodied. Although the dualistic separation of consciousness from body that underlies transmigration is retained within the VHP, as highlighted by the fact that Jernigan, despite his antisocial deviance during life, is posthumously touted to be an exemplar of anatomical normality, the precise form in which post-biological "life" continues is thus upturned. The VHs, as resurrected digital entities, exemplify Moravec's concept of the post-biological in a very literal sense; they exist beyond the parameters of human life. Applying the term "post-biological" to the VH bodies is thus somewhat ironic; undoubtedly the VHs exist beyond their biological lifetimes, but where this posthumous existence in Moravec's scenario is posited to be consciousness, within the VHP, it is instead a post-biological (and virtual) corporeality. Jernigan and the Maryland housewife are corporeally resurrected as post-biological entities, existing eternally within the virtual realm.

Hence, the primary ontological transformation enacted by the VHP occurs through the digitization of bodies, both actually and conceptually. At a material level, the body is literally transmogrified into digital information when the physical body of the corpse is disintegrated and transformed into the VH's digital body. The transformation of the physical body within the VHP is also concomitant with a conceptual reordering of human flesh that permeates the project in a wider sense; the anatomical body, both in the form of the VH, and in other bodies generally, is reconfigured in accordance with the principles of the digital. Visual theorist William J. Mitchell, in *The Reconfigured Eye*, elucidates the fragmentary tendency of the digital by comparing chemical and digital photography.[11] He suggests that the digital image, no matter how high its resolution, is necessarily comprised of pixels; while these reconstructed pixels in the form of a photograph might resemble an analogue image, the digital image is nonetheless derived from individual segments and, subsequently, can never be completely seamless.[12] The VH bodies, comprised as they are of a sequence of digital images, reflect this fragmentary logic at a compositional level, as does the body of the VM in *BodyVoyage*.

The reconfiguration of materiality in accordance with the digital fragment is further evinced in the VHP's fragmentation of the body into discrete values; the VHs are fragmented, not just informatically in terms of their digital composition, but also through the geometric segmentation of the body. That is, the VH body is comprised of discrete values rather than continuous flesh, through its geometric composition, segmented at 1mm or 0.3mm intervals.[13] This perception of the body as comprised of discrete fragments within the VHP indicates a conceptual departure from the compartmentalized body of traditional anatomy, where the body's various layers and organs are peeled away to reveal further layers below. Cultural theorists Eugene Thacker and José van Dijck, in their respective essays on the VHP, draw attention to the significance of this transformation, noting that the anatomical body shifts from being conceptually partitioned in accordance with its anatomical structures, such as organs, and is instead constituted as a series of planar images.[14] In this way, the representational mode of the VHP, with its geometric delineations of bodily space, departs from anatomical illustrations that simulate three-dimensional depth using linear perspective.[15] As Neal Curtis explains, the particular mode of reconfiguring the body that occurs within the VHP does not reflect an innate physical reality of the human body, but is rather derived from anatomical ideology.[16] The VH, then, is not a neutral representation of the anatomical body, but rather the model for a particular kind of body produced by the intersection of anatomy and digital technologies. Moreover, the logic underpinning the VHP extends, by implication, to the "normal" bodies of which the VHs are allegedly representative. From this, the reconfiguration of the material body within the VHP is concomitant with a broader conceptual transformation of human ontology through the creation of a post-biological entity. As will be discussed, the consequences of this post-biological ontology are revealed by an analysis of the tropes of horror and nostalgia that permeate both the VHP and *BodyVoyage*.

As a means for further elaborating the ontological imaginings of post-biological life, it is worth considering a peculiar reference in the introduction to Tsiaras's *BodyVoyage* book, which is based upon the CD-ROM. In the introduction to the book, John Hockenberry writes that Tsiaras has achieved "a sense of art and tranquillity worthy of a da Vinci. He has achieved it by using the virtual methodology of an ancient Egyptian embalmer or a digital Jeffrey Dahmer."[17] This strange description highlights two particular cultural economies at work within both the VHP itself and the *BodyVoyage* program. The reference to embalmment is suggestive of the project's desire to preserve, and indeed resurrect, an intact, integrated human body beyond death. Yet the very process of preservation, which takes the form of digitization in the VHP, radically changes both the material status and the appearance of the body that is preserved, rendering the original intact body irretrievable. The impossible desire to resurrect an intact, original body within the virtual realm is suggestive of a nostalgic longing for the possibility of recreating an "authentic" body in vitro. This longing is intertwined with the radical disintegration of bodily integrity that occurs in the transmogrification process: The horror of these bodily mutilations, as suggested by the reference to the serial killer Jeffrey Dahmer, means that the post-biological entity can never be fully invested with the authenticity or integrity that is lost during the resurrection process. These modes of horror and nostalgia that arise from the VHP and *BodyVoyage* are elicited as viewer/reader responses through the framing and representation of the VH bodies, and it is to these modalities that this discussion will now turn.

## POST-BIOLOGICAL HORROR: THE BODY DISINTEGRATED

One of the most bizarre and explicit references to horror within *BodyVoyage* occurs, as noted, in Tsiaras's book, where John Hockenberry compares Tsiaras with Jeffrey Dahmer.[18] This comparison between Tsiaras and one of the United States' most notorious and publicized serial killers is incongruous, to say the least.[19] Dahmer was a necrophiliac cannibal who murdered seventeen men; such a comparison is hardly flattering to Tsiaras. Yet there are notable parallels between Dahmer's treatment of his victims and the VHP's treatment of the bodies of Jernigan and the Maryland housewife. Dahmer dismembered and then photographed the corpses of his victims before storing various body parts in his apartment. At the time of his arrest, he had one victim's head in the refrigerator and three heads stored in the freezer, in addition to numerous other body parts scattered throughout his abode.[20] The peculiar comparison to Dahmer in *BodyVoyage* might therefore be explained by the remarkable similarities between the treatment of the VH bodies and that of Dahmer's victims; in both cases, bodies were dismembered, photographed, and then frozen. The comparison made between Tsiaras and Dahmer would seem to suggest that, while the VHP is a far more sanitized and clinical replication of the body-mutilations carried out by Dahmer, the horror evoked by Dahmer's actions nonetheless haunts the VHP.[21]

From one perspective, this instance of horror within the VHP might be understood in relation to Thacker's model of "biohorror." Thacker uses the term to explain the particular horror that results from the reframing of the body by technoscience.[22] According to Thacker, biohorror considers

> [w]hat it would mean to take the human body, and, through a set of procedures and techniques, transform that body into something non-human (posthuman, inhuman), into something that implicitly transgresses the biological, anthropomorphic, and evolutionary traditions of defining the human.[23]

As Thacker explains, biohorror derives from the manifestations of science and technology upon the body of a subject; the resulting sense of horror is a consequence of the disjunction between human embodiment and technological transformations of the body.[24] This conceptualization of biohorror renders it applicable to a wide range of contexts in which "horror," in one form or another, arises from human-technoscientific interaction. While biohorror is thus a useful means for considering these interactions in a generalist sense, the flexibility of this term means that it does not necessarily account for the specific horror elicited by the digital resurrection of the VHs.

To this end, "post-biological horror" takes into consideration the particularities of both the VHP and *BodyVoyage*, pertaining to the geometric disintegration and digital reintegration of the VHs.[25] Post-biological horror may be described as the affect elicited by the complete decimation of the body's organic form and the reordering of its physicality in terms of geometric rather than organic principles. Where many theorists emphasize the fleshiness, disorder, and viscerality of the horrific body, the horror of the post-biological body results from precisely the opposite reason. The absolute fleshlessness and geometric rigidity of the VH body constitute the basis for the horror it elicits. This reformulation of horror, in terms of the post-biological, is markedly different from the model of horror forwarded by well-known theorists such as Barbara Creed and Julia Kristeva. Within such psychoanalytically derived models, horror is often understood in relation to the capacity of the disordered body to defile and threaten the symbolic order.[26] According to this paradigm, the body of horror is typically excessive, visceral, and fluid.[27] Yet, as will be revealed, the digitality of the VHs renders void many of these characteristics of the horrific because of the VHs' absence of tangible corporeality.

Even without its being mutilated and digested as Dahmer's victims were, the VH body within psychoanalytic discourse would be perceived as horrific simply because of its status as corpse. Kristeva writes that the corpse, "seen without God [...] is the utmost of abjection," suggesting that it is imbued with an innate sense of horror. [28] As she explains, the fundamental horror of the corpse results from its capacity as "a border that has encroached upon everything" to symbolize the dissolution of order.[29] Following this logic, it would seem that the VH's embodiment of horror derives at least in part from being created from a corpse. Yet, while the VH corpses and their posthumous dissection are recounted in detail in descriptions of the VHP, the process of death itself, its messiness and viscerality, is left conspicuously absent in such accounts. On the NLM's VHP Web page, for example, very few details are given about the VF's death, other than that she "willed her body to science," while the institutional murder of the VM is described cursorily.[30] Likewise, the death of Jernigan is described only briefly in *BodyVoyage*:

> [T]he drugs began flowing at 12:23AM. [Jernigan] coughed quickly six times, his head and shoulders jerking with each cough, and was pronounced dead eight minuteslater. The Texas anatomical board took custody of the body, and it was flown to Spitzer and Whitlock's laboratory in Denver.[31]

Perhaps the most telling aspect of this clinical description of death is the eight minutes between Jernigan's coughs and the pronunciation of his death, which are condensed into a single sentence. This cursoriness is made particularly apparent when comparing the description of Jernigan's death to that of his posthumous dissection. The "Introduction" in *BodyVoyage* gives a detailed description of the process of dissection, from the freezing and segmentation to the slicing and imaging of his body, all with the graphic detail that is absent in the descriptions of his death. Through this, the horror of death in the VHP is erased, its significance annulled, such that death becomes merely a brief transitionary phase in the transmogrification from living body to digital body. Likewise, the VHP's sanitized images of the interior lack the viscerality of the body cleft open as described by Kristeva. Users of the VH dataset are spared the messy and unpleasant procedure of "real" dissection by manipulating the VH data electronically.[32] The grotesque sensory qualities of the anatomical cadaver are similarly annulled in the VH bodies through their transformation into digital entities; there is no wetness of blood, no smell of formaldehyde, no squelch of severed flesh.[33] In the same way that death in the VHP is reconceived as a clinical act, devoid of horror, so too is the VH body, through its transmogrification into virtual body, purged of such horrific or grotesque qualities as wetness or incontainability.

Where the theorization of classical horror does not adequately explain the grisliness particular to the VHP, post-biological horror proves to be a useful concept for theorizing the form of body horror particular to the VH bodies. Rather than the visceral and fleshy bodies of horror described by Kristeva and Creed, the body of post-biological horror is characterized by its reconfiguration of bodily order according to abstract geometric (rather than organic) principles. The horror evoked by the VHs relates to their transmogrification into entities that, while existing virtually, are devoid of organic materiality. This post-biological horror in the VHP occurs in two main ways. First, at a material level, through the cryosectioning process, the VH body is reordered according to a geometric order, and with this reordering the body loses its imagined organic integrity. Second, the reordering of the body enacts a reconfiguration of corporeality, wherein the digital body exists as an informatic entity, devoid of substance and humanity.

The geometrizing aspect of post-biological horror is particularly evident in the grisly description of the process used to create the VM, as detailed in *Atlas of the Visible Male*.[34] Spitzer and Whitlock describe the process of sawing the VM body, noting that "[n]o actual slices were retained [...] since we destroyed each documented slice by milling it down to get to the one underneath."[35] The use of the verb "mill" in this description has a particularly gruesome undertone, suggestive of the milling of a body as if it were a block of wood being fed into a wood-chipper.[36] While the horror of this particular dissection of the body recalls Creed's notion of the body-horror of mutilation, it also reveals a further horror particular to the VHP; this description does not simply evoke a horror of dismemberment generally, but also a horror pertaining specifically to the geometric segmentation of the body. This geometrizing occurs both physically, with the actual sawing of the body, and conceptually, in the reconfiguration of the body as a gridded object capable of being transformed into discrete values.

Indeed, Catherine Waldby, in her extensive study of the VHP, writes of the reconfiguration of the body that occurs within the VHP, suggesting that it registers the body's "spatial organisation as a registered (that is, gridded in three dimensions–xyz) geometric volume."[37] This geometric conceptualization of the body that occurs within the VHP is in stark contrast to the partitioning conceptualization of the body in the context of anatomical dissection. Anatomical dissection undoubtedly constitutes a form of horrific bodily dismemberment, as Katherine Young has shown in her study of the grotesque body of anatomical evisceration.[38] Yet, unlike the milling of the VM, anatomical dissection, with its careful evisceration and compartmentalization of the body's organs, partitions the body according to a kind of "natural" order; that is, it is mutilated according to its own internal structure, such that while the gross integrity of the body is destroyed, its individual components remain largely intact.

Any notion of a "natural" order underlying the physical body is necessarily problematic, as the organ-based compartmentalization of the body is no more "natural" than a Galenic order of the body's four humors.[39] Yet despite this, organic compartmentalization has a material reality that is visible to the dissector or anatomist, whether it be individual organs or different tissue types. In contrast, the indiscriminate dissection by "milling" of the VH body violates the corporeal order by reconfiguring the body as comprised of uniform segments that bear no relation to its overall, and visible, organic structure.[40] It is precisely this reordering of the body in accordance with a geometrical model that evokes the affect of horror in response to the "milling" and shaving of the body.[41] In this context, the body is not treated like an anatomical cadaver, where the structure of either the living or the inanimate body informs its posthumous mutilation, but rather, is rendered as an inanimate, inorganic object, analogous to a block of wood able to be chipped into uniform segments. This reconfiguration of the body indicates a crucial aspect of the VHP; the corpse is perceived to be object rather than subject. The use of a saw to "mill" the VHP corpses renders, in many ways, the connection between the living body and the corpse void. Thus, the mechanistic mutilation of the body in the VHP symbolically shatters the imagined integrity of the corporeal body; through its transmogrification into a virtual body, whose primary principle of order is geometric rather than organic, the body is rendered as inorganic object.

One of the key aspects of the post-biological horror of the VHP is thus the physical and conceptual geometrizing of the corpse into a nonhuman object, transforming it into an entity vastly different from a living body. The segmentation of the body that occurs through this process is mirrored in the further transposition of that body into digital information. Where the geometrized body of the VH is spatially compartmentalized according to a three-dimensional grid, the segmentation that occurs from this is enhanced by the translation of this grid into digital information. This is particularly apparent in the different modes of visualizing the VH body in the *BodyVoyage* program. In all the various modules of the program, including animations and cross-sections, hyperbright images of the VM float ghost-like upon a black background, framed by a grid that gives the illusion of three-dimensional space (Fig. 6.1) In the gallery mode, for example, users can view individual bodily sections, which are partitioned according to the four segments in which the VM was originally chopped: head, torso, pelvis, and legs. The central image of the chosen bodily fragment—for example, the head—is animated so that it appears, chameleon-like, to change color every second, moving back and forth between states of opacity and transparency as it slowly spins around. The turning fragment is also framed by the grid that recurs throughout the program. This grid that surrounds the pulsing image of the bodily fragment geometrizes the imagined space in which the body floats, echoing the geometric segmentation of the VH corpse and imbuing the virtual body with a simulated corporeal depth. Each gridded square recalls not only the geometric disintegration of the corpse but also its digital reintegration. Likewise, the hundreds of tiny squares mimic the subsequent pixellation of the body after its digital manipulation. What is horrific in the gallery of *Body-Voyage* is not simply the fact of geometric mutilation but also post-biological existence itself: the radical disintegration of the body actually and conceptually underlies the horror evoked by this representation of virtual humanity.

The ghoulish sense of horror elicited by *BodyVoyage* thus derives in part from the horror of a posthumous corporeal existence. This resonates with the horror elicited by the mutilation of the corpse, as evident in the metaphor of cannibalism suggested by Hockenberry's reference to Dahmer. Part of the horror of Dahmer's crime resulted from the way in which his treatment of victims rendered their corpses analogous to digestible meat; like the VHP's mechanistic sawing of the VH corpses, the body in this scenario is disintegrated, both actually and conceptually. This reconfiguration of the corpse as object is radically removed from the act of preservation that seeks to maintain corporeal integrity beyond death. The VHP, despite disintegrating the corpse, paradoxically incorporates this element of preservation by resurrecting the body. Within the VHP and *BodyVoyage*, there is fundamental contradiction: At same time that the project enacts a horrific geometrizing bodily mutilation, it aims to preserve the integrity of the corpse within a virtual realm.

## POST-BIOLOGICAL NOSTALGIA: PRESERVING
## THE AUTHENTIC BODY

To return to the comparison in the *BodyVoyage* book between Tsiaras and an "ancient Egyptian embalmer," it would seem that the post-biological nostalgia of both the VHP and *BodyVoyage* resonates with the fraught tension that underlies human preservation. Embalmment has at its core an impossible desire to continue the appearance of life beyond death. Likewise, the VHP seeks to reinvest death with life by virtually resurrecting the corpse and proclaiming its heavily mediated digital incarnation as anatomically authentic. In *BodyVoyage*, this desire is taken further; the images in the program and in the book involve a large amount of remediation, such as the retinting of the colors of the VH body to make it appear more spectacular. As noted earlier, the project's problematic claim to represent "authentic" human anatomy by presenting the mediated body of the VM is illustrated by the grid in *BodyVoyage*. This grid appears to reassure the viewer of the original three-dimensionality of Jernigan's body, as if to emphasize that, despite its current existence as data projected onto a screen, Jernigan's body once had a material reality. The irony of presenting this digital body as if it were "real," and somehow unmodified, is highlighted in the Gallery module of the *BodyVoyage* program (Fig. 6.3). The series of small images superimposed on the grid is highlighted by simulated up-lighting, rendering them analogous to photographs in an art gallery. The way in which these images frame the pulsing bodily fragment in the center, with its simulated spatial depth, suggests that, while the small images are precisely that—images—the animated body in the center is somehow more "real" or "alive" than the images surrounding it.

This desire to simulate an "authentic" or "real" body within the realm of the virtual underlies the concept of post-biological nostalgia. Post-biological nostalgia can be identified in the VHP in three ways. First, the project exhibits a nostalgic desire for a body unmediated by technology, evident in the requirement for the VH bodies to be free of techno-surgical modification. Second, the requisition of the VH bodies as ideal, anatomically normative specimens indicates a further longing for an impossibly ideal body that is anatomically representative of all bodies. Finally, this desire for normativity, when coupled with the capacity of the VH bodies to be endlessly manipulated, regenerated, and resurrected, as in *BodyVoyage*, signals a longing for all human bodies to be as malleable and renewable as the VHs.

One of the crucial selection criteria for the VH bodies was that they be devoid of any evidence of interventional surgery or technology, including artificial joints, prostheses, or pacemakers. The iteration of the VHP's key criteria for a normative anatomical specimen as unmediated by technological intervention seems strangely at odds with the complex technologizing of the body that occurred during the process of creating the VHs. Such a tension signals an anxiety about the authenticity of the anatomical body, and with it, a longing for the possibility of a body unmediated by technology. Within the VHP, and within *BodyVoyage*, this longing takes the form of a nostalgia for an idealized, pretechnological body. Post-biological nostalgia in this context signifies an unfulfillable longing for an organically authentic body that permeates narratives of the synthetic resurrection of the VHs.

Nostalgia arguably denotes a sense of sadness derived from the longing for an object or place from the past.[42] This notion of the imagined past as the foundation for nostalgia might be considered in relation to the body of the VHs. David Ellison, in his study of the VHP, describes the basis for this nostalgia, noting that:

> We live in an era of prosthetics, of miniaturized machines beneath the skin. The dream vision of the VHP undoes this, sends us back to a moment innocent of hip replacements, pacemakers, metal pins, and internal monitors. This quaintly romantic body, frozen in time and gelatin, is then offered as a blank slate for the computer mouse to manipulate.[43]

Thus, the VHs, with their anachronistically unprostheticized anatomy, recall an imagined past wherein bodies existed in an anatomically unaltered state. Through its insistence that the normative body of the VH be free of technological intervention, the VHP essentially seeks to resurrect a medically pure body, untainted by technological intervention or modification. Such a longing signals a desire to reinstate the possibility of anatomical "authenticity," uncorrupted by technology. Where the dream of transmigration described by Moravec centers on human evolution intertwined with technology, ironically, the realization of post-biological existence in the VHP is fraught with an anxious insistence about returning to a pretechnological purity of the body.

Through this desire, the VHP is invested with an anxiety about the ultimate impossibility of the idealized body for which it longs. The inauthentic "past" that is sought by the VHP, in the form of a pretechnological body, is impossible to retrieve; despite the VHP claiming to represent a body unaltered by medical technology, all representations of the VHs are, ironically, necessarily mediated by digital technology. The physical bodies of the VHs, as they are completely disintegrated, can never again be viewed in the flesh or in their entirety, but can only be decoded from digital data and reimaged through the mediating interface of the computer screen. It would seem that, despite its insistent longing for an "authentic," pretechnological body as a normative ideal, the VHP is simultaneously invested with an anxiety that such a category might in fact be obsolete.

This longing for an authentic body within the VHP can be understood by considering Louis J. Kern's notion of the elusiveness of the "natural" body. As Kern describes, the large number of surgical and technological modifications enacted on the body in modern culture, such as cosmetic surgery, organ transplants, and neuro-prosthetic implants, results in a significant diminishment of human individuals who could be considered "natural."[44] As he suggests, many technologies of body modification are founded on an assumption about the inherent imperfection and corruption of the human body.[45] In light of this, the VHP's nostalgia for a pretechnological body becomes symptomatic of a wider cultural anxiety about the impossibility of an anatomically "natural" body; not only is a nontechnologized body an elusive object, but the very concept of such a body is fraught with an anxiety that it is inherently imperfect and incomplete. In this context, the post-biological nostalgia of the VHP centers a paradoxical desire.

There is a further instance of post-biological nostalgia that occurs within the VHP and also pertains to the impossible longing for an anatomically normative body. This is particularly apparent in the process undertaken in the VHP to obtain suitable bodies to be the VM and the VF. As the project's creators Victor Spitzer and David Whitlock note, their "most formidable task was to locate a specimen that could be taken as 'normal' or representative of a large population."[46] The difficulty experienced by the NLM in obtaining a viable specimen of normal anatomy reveals the arbitrariness of normalizing anatomy: Out of six thousand bodies, Jernigan, despite having only one testicle and lacking both a number fourteen tooth and an appendix, was nonetheless the best available exemplar of "normal" anatomy that could be obtained. As Ellison points out, this difficulty arises in part from the fact that an anatomically "normal" cadaver is anything but "normal"; that is, people usually die of either illness or trauma, thus rendering them either pathologically or physically abnormal, and hence unrepresentative of the general population.[47]

The ability to obtain a healthy and "normal" cadaver—that is, from a body killed neither by illness nor trauma—for use in the VHP was thus possible largely because of the legitimization of capital punishment in the United States.[48] From this, it is ironic that Jernigan's body, in the form of the VH, exists as an alleged exemplar of anatomical normality only because of the extraordinariness of his crime.[49] Likewise, Jernigan's well-developed musculature, which further added to his suitability as a normative specimen, was not as the result of any "normal" development but was rather exaggerated from years of lifting weights while in prison. Thus, the VHP's

longing for the possibility of an idealized anatomical body, a perfect specimen representative of humanity, is tainted by the impossibility of achieving
this desire. Where nostalgia constitutes "pangs of longing for another time,
another place, another self," the longed-for, imagined self in the VHP is an
idealized model of anatomical normality, one that is nonexistent in "reality," but that is reimagined within the VHP.[50] Subsequently, the post-biological nostalgia of the VHP is founded on a discontinuity between modes
of normalcy and pathology, where the anatomically normative body of the
VH, as the object of nostalgic desire, is, by definition, abnormal.

   This tension between a longed-for model of normality in the extraordinary body of the VH parallels the VHP's creation of an "authentic" body
that is capable of endless regeneration and resurrection, particularly in its
manifestation in *BodyVoyage*. Ashraf Aziz and James McKenzie, in their
plea for the virtues of "real" anatomical cadavers over digital cadavers for
anatomical instruction, note the unrepresentativeness of digital cadavers,
describing their use in medical education as founded on an inaccurate
assumption that "the human body is a monolithic, abstract entity."[51] Unlike
"real" cadavers, they claim, digital cadavers are not representative of
"normal" bodies; they not only lack the physicality encountered in real
bodies, but also have a quality of invariability.[52] The VH body, with its
capacity to be digitally dismantled and reintegrated in its original form, has
a similar capacity for endlessly reiterated truth.[53] This is particularly evident
in *BodyVoyage*, where the VM can be repeatedly disintegrated in the various
modules of the program (head/torso/thighs/legs) and then reintegrated in
the "Whole Body Viewer" section. Indeed, this would seem to fulfil
Spitzer's and Whitlock's claim that "we now have a renewable cadaver, a
standardized patient, and a basis for digital populations of the future. Not
only can we dissect it, we can put it back together again and start all over."[54]

   Concurrent with this wish to reconstruct the mutilated body of the
cadaver is the desire for a living patient body that is similarly as mutable
and reliable as a virtual one. The VH is thus presented as an ideal body to
which other human bodies should aspire, not only in terms of its anatomical structure, but also in relation to its quality of reversibility. This signals a
desire for control over bodily aberrance that is inherent in the VHP's
anatomical enterprise; where the ideal cadaver, like the ideal "standardized
patient" is a fixed and accountable body, the uncontrollable body is, by
implication, anatomically inferior, if not "abnormal." This concern again
highlights the condition of post-biological nostalgia where technological
transformation of the body is concomitant with a desire to preserve its
alleged authenticity.

   The VHP and its products such as *BodyVoyage* incorporate a fundamental tension that forms the basis for post-biological horror and nostal-

gia. On the one hand, the VHP reiterates a technophilic model of post-biological life, wherein the physical body is a discardable, imperfect vessel, and the digital body is eminently superior in terms of its malleability and capacity for renewal. Yet simultaneously, through the process of transmogrification, the VHP and *BodyVoyage* attempt to reinstate the importance of corporeality by resurrecting a pretechnological, "authentic" body. The VHs' embodiment of these contradictory elements highlights the radical reconfiguration of human corporeality that occurs with post-biological ontology. The VHs simultaneously embody both corporeal integrity and corporeal dissolution. The very act of preservation, in the form of digital embalmment, is thus shadowed by the radical disintegration of the body that is necessary in order to maintain post-biological life. Horror and nostalgia are thus intertwined in the post-biological ontology enacted by digital transmogrification.

## NOTES

1. Alexander Tsiaras, *BodyVoyage*. CD-ROM. Time Warner Publishing, 1997a.

2. See Csordas for a discussion of the significance, in a Foucauldian sense, of the increased surveillance of the female body compared to the male. Thomas J. Csordas, "Computerized Cadavers: Shades of Being and Representation in Virtual Reality," in *Biotechnology and Culture: Bodies, Anxieties, Ethics*, ed. Paul E. Brodwin (Bloomington: Indiana University Press, 2000).

3. National Library of Medicine, *Visible Human Project Gallery*, http://www.nlm.nih.gov/research/visible/mpeg/umd_video.mpg, accessed March 7, 2007.

4. The NLM Web site (http://www.nlm.nih.gov/research/visible/products.html) lists dozens of projects, mostly anatomically educational, that have been derived from the VH datasets. The dataset has also been used for filmic special effects, such as the reincarnation of LeeLu's body in Luc Besson's film, *The Fifth Element*, directed by Luc Besson (Columbia Pictures, 1997).

5. David Ellison, "Anatomy of a Murderer," *21.C* 3 (1995): 20-25, 24.

6. Ibid., 24.

7. Given the rapid development of computer technologies in the last decade, this problem will no doubt diminish. As the capacity of computer memory increases, the size of the VH datasets will increasingly become less of an obstacle to members of the general public who wish to download it.

8. Tsiaras has also published a book entitled *BodyVoyage: A Three-Dimensional Tour of a Real Human Body*; filled with spectacular images and virtually no written information, it is more like a lavishly illustrated coffee-table tome than an anatomical textbook. For the purposes of this chapter, I will focus predominantly on the

*BodyVoyage* CD-ROM; future references to *BodyVoyage* in this chapter will denote the CD-ROM, unless specified otherwise.

9. Hans Moravec, *Mind Children: The Future of Robot and Human Intelligence* (Cambridge: Harvard University Press, 1988), 108-09.

10. This peculiar and unique ontology seems at first glance commensurate with the posthuman. Certainly, in relation to N. Katherine Hayles's understanding of the posthuman as predicated on a capacity for human-machine synthesis, it would seem that the bodies of the VHs have indeed been perfectly aligned with digital technology. Yet the posthuman predominantly imagines the "human" to be one intrinsically connected with subjectivity and selfhood. That is, the human "self" that is integrated with the machine is almost invariably one with consciousness, where this consciousness, as it is interrogated by Hayles, may be either embodied or disembodied. In contrast, the resurrected "self" of the VHP is completely corporeal, despite the project's inclinations toward mind-body dualism. See N. Katherine Hayles, *How We Became Posthuman: Virtual Bodies in Cybernetics, Literature, and Informatics* (Chicago: University of Chicago Press, 1999).

11. William J. Mitchell, *The Reconfigured Eye: Visual Truth in the Post-Photographic Era* (Cambridge: MIT Press, 1992), 5.

12. Ibid., 5.

13. Ibid., 5. As Catherine Waldby describes this situation, "[a]s digital photographs, the VH data exist not as continuous field of shade variation, the non-quantifiable, analogue surface of seamless gradations which is the photograph, but rather as a discrete grid of image elements." Catherine Waldby, *The Visible Human Project: Informatic Bodies and Posthuman Medicine* (London: Routledge, 2000), 100.

14. José Van Dijck, *The Transparent Body: A Cultural Analysis of Medical Imaging* (Seattle: University of Washington Press, 2005), 124. Van Dijck notes that this reconceptualization of the body in "slices rather than pieces" mirrors the increasing use within modern medicine of imaging technologies to view the body-interior; this mode of "reading" the VH corpses is thus congruent with the way in which the living body is "read" in diagnostic medicine. Likewise, Eugene Thacker writes that in the VHP, "The partitioning logic of modern anatomy [...] has been abandoned [...]. Instead, with a view towards digital-visual media and the Internet, the body of the VHP is reconstituted along the lines of scanning and surface data most appropriate for digital image processing and digital file standardization." Eugene Thacker, ".../Visible_Human.Html/ Digital Anatomy and the Hyper-Texted Body," *CTheory* a060, http://www.ctheory. net/printer.asp?id=103.

15. It is useful here to distinguish between the representational techniques used in the VH dataset and the traditional anatomical textbook. Illustrations in traditional anatomy textbooks represent the body's anatomy as it is revealed by dissection. Écorché series, for example, mimic the gradual peeling away and exposition of

anatomical layers during dissection. This form of representation accords with the medical gaze as it is defined by Michel Foucault. The anatomical illustration depicts physical volume using the representative technique of linear perspective, and, in doing so, mimics the way in which the body's physical volume is perceived by the anatomist or physician. Michel Foucault, *The Birth of the Clinic: An Archaeology of Medical Perception*, trans. A. M.Sheridan Smith (London: Tavistock, 1973), 135-36.

16. Neal Curtis, "The Body as Outlaw: Lyotard, Kafka and the Visible Human Project," *Body & Society* 5, nos. 2-3 (1999), 261. Curtis writes: "The VHP reproduces not a 'complete' body as it would have us believe, but the body as perceived by the particular discourse of which it is a product."

17. John Hockenberry, introduction to *BodyVoyage: A Three-Dimensional Tour of a Real Human Body*, by Alexander Tsiaras (New York: Warner Books, 1997).

18. Ibid.

19. In fact, this is not the only reference to Jeffery Dahmer in press releases concerning the VHP. In *Atlas of the Visible Human Male*, Spitzer and Whitlock write of their concern about reactions to the VHP's initial press release, and their subsequent relief when any negative press about the VHP was overshadowed by a far more gruesome headline reading "Cannibal Dahmer Killed in Jail." Spitzer and Whitlock seem to imply that, while the VHP seems gruesome and perhaps morally questionable, it is, relative to other incidences of death and bodily violation, ethically mild. Victor M. Spitzer and David G. Whitlock, *Atlas of the Visible Human Male: Reverse Engineering of the Human Body* (Boston: Jones & Bartlett, 1998), xvii.

20. http://www.bbc.co.uk/crime/caseclosed/dahmer1.shtml

21. For an in-depth discussion of the VHP in relation to haunting, see CatherineWaldby, *The Visible Human Project: Informatic Bodies and Posthuman Medicine*, 136-56.

22. Eugene Thacker, "Biohorror/Biotech," *Paradoxa: Studies in World Literary Genres* 17 (2002), 109.

23. Ibid., 116-17.

24. Ibid., 113.

25. For a discussion of horror in relation to nanotechnology, see Colin Milburn, "Nano/Splatter: Disintegrating the Postbiological Body," *New Literary History* 36, no. 2 (2005), 283-311.

26. Julia Kristeva, *Powers of Horror: An Essay on Abjection*, trans. Leon S. Roudiez (New York: Columbia University Press, 1982), 3-4; Barbara Creed, "Horror and the Carnivalesque," in *Fields of Vision: Essays in Film Studies, Visual Anthropology, and Photography*, ed. Leslie Devereaux and Roger Hillman (Berkeley: University of California Press, 1995), 145, 149.

27. Kristeva, *Powers of Horror*, 3; Creed, "Horror and the Carnivalesque," 150.

28. Kristeva, *Powers of Horror*, 4.

29. Ibid., 3.

30. National Library of Medicine, "Marching through the Visible Man," http://www.nlm.nih.gov/research/visible/vhp_conf/lorensen/vm/vm.htm, accessed March 7, 2007, and National Library of Medicine, "Marching through the Visible Woman," http://www.nlm. nih.gov/research/visible/vhp_conf/ lorensen/vw/vw.htm, accessed March 7, 2007.

31. Jeff Goldberg, "Introduction," in *BodyVoyage* by Alexander Tsiaras. CD-ROM. Time Warner Publishing, 1997a.

32. Cartwright, "A Cultural Anatomy of the Visible Human Project," in *The Visible Woman: Imaging Technologies, Gender, and Science*, eds. Paula A. Treichler, Lisa Cartwright and Constance Penley (New York: New York University Press, 1998), 27.

33. Indeed, just as users are spared the gory task of dissecting a real cadaver by manipulating the virtual body of the VH, this would seem to be similarly the case for the creators of the VHP. It would appear that they, too, because of their $5000 backsaw and the capacity to freeze the VH bodies, avoided the wet evisceration of a traditional dissection. Yet, despite access to such advanced technology, the duration of cutting sessions was often restricted by environmental factors, specifically the lack of air-conditioning in the laboratory in which the procedure took place; that is, during the cutting sessions, the body began to thaw. The irony of this situation does not escape Spitzer and Whitlock, who note that, despite the massive technological process involved in the VHP, "we were still somewhat limited by refrigeration, one of the same constraints encountered by fifteenth-century anatomists." Thus, despite the apparent sanitization of the dissection process by rendering the body clean and dry through freezing, the body's innate wetness, its viscerality, nonetheless inhibited the cryosectioning process. Spitzer and Whitlock, *Atlas of the Visible Human Male*, xvi.

34. Ibid., p. 6.

35. Ibid., p. 6.

36. Indeed, the term "mill," when considered in the context of milling flour, has further connotations with the metaphor of cannibalism invoked in *BodyVoyage*.

37. Waldby, *The Visible Human Project*, 72.

38. Anatomical dissection, as Katharine Young points out, "incises fresh cuts, slits, apertures into the body [, and therefore] the dissected body is a grotesque body." Katharine Young, "Still Life with Corpse: Management of the Grotesque Body in Medicine" in *Bodylore,* ed. Katharine Young (Knoxville: University of Tennessee Press, 1993), 114.

39. Foucault, *The Birth of the Clinic*, 127. The social and cultural bases underlying such conceptualizations of the body are illustrated in Michel Foucault's discussion of the medical gaze. For a discussion of the cultural logics underpinning human dissection, see Jonathan Sawday, *The Body Emblazoned: Dissection and the Human Body in Renaissance Culture* (London: Routledge, 1995).

40. As Thacker describes this, the "partitioning logic of modern anatomy, whereby the body whole is hierarchically broken down into integrated physiological systems (circulatory, respiratory, muscular, reproductive, etc.), organs, tissues, and cells— that logic has been abandoned in the production [...] of the Visible Man. [...] the body of the VHP is reconstituted along the lines of scanning and surface data most appropriate for digital image processing." Thacker, "...／Visible_ Human.Html/Digital Anatomy and the Hypter-Texted Body."

41. This "milling" the body by shaving slices off it evokes images of a commercial slicer used to shave a leg of ham or to slice cheese, and in this way recalls the reference to cannibalism implicit in the comparison between Tsiaras and Dahmer. Indeed, the trope of cannibalism is further evident in Spitzer and Whitlock's book corresponding to the VM, *Atlas of the Visible Human Male*. In the book's introduction, as a means for illustrating how the body is visualized in its transverse, coronal and sagittal planes, the book depicts a banana sliced in corresponding planes. Not only is the banana sliced in its anatomical planes, but these slices are also depicted as culinary photographs, looking far more like the pages of a 1950s cookbook than a late-twentieth-century, highly technologized anatomical textbook. The banana slices in the transverse plane are displayed on top of a bowl of breakfast cereal, possibly rice bubbles, the coronally sliced banana sits atop a cake, and the sagittally carved banana frames a mound of ice cream in what appears to be a banana split. Sadly, and perhaps due to a lack of culinary imagination on the part of the book's authors, the bananas sliced along their oblique and curved planes are not afforded any culinary setting whatsoever, but appear only on a black background. Aside from the obvious sexual connotations of using a phallic banana to signify the male body, the comparison between human anatomy and food is somewhat telling. Specifically, the use of a banana, as a soft peelable fruit, to signify the body seems particularly appropriate for a discipline concerned primarily with the visualization of subcutaneous structures. In addition, the comparative easiness of slicing up a banana compared to slicing a complete human body suggests that the ideal body of the VM, once in digital form, can be broken down into slices as easily as cutting a piece of fruit. Unlike the messy, unpleasant, and complicated procedure of dissecting a real human body, the VH can be dissected as easily and as free of gore as preparing breakfast; no longer exclusively relegated to the domain of the clinic, the anatomical body can now be manipulated and digested at home.

42. As Susan Stewart describes nostalgia, it is "a sadness without an object, a sadness which creates a longing that of necessity is inauthentic because it does not take part in lived experience. Rather, it remains behind and before that experience. Nostalgia, like any form of narrative, is always ideological: the past it seeks has

never existed except as narrative, and hence, always absent, that past continually threatens to reproduce itself as a felt lack." Susan Stewart, *On Longing: Narratives of the Miniature, the Gigantic, the Souvenir, the Collection* (Baltimore: John Hopkins University Press, 1984), 23.

43. Ellison, "Anatomy of a Murderer," 25.

44. Louis J. Kern, "Terminal Notions of What We May Become: Synthflesh, Cyberreality, and the Post-Human Body," in *Simulacrum America: The USA and the Popular Media,* ed. Elisabeth Kraus and Carolin Auer (New York: Camden House, 2000), 98.

45. Kern writes: "The human body has increasingly been modified by electronic implants to regulate somatic functions, cosmetic surgery, organ transplants, and neuro-prosthetic devices. A significant portion of the human community can no longer be classified as purely 'natural.' Indeed, body alteration is rooted in a consciousness of the imperfection, the corruption of human flesh." Kern, "Terminal Notions," 98.

46. Spitzer and Whitlock, *Atlas of the Visible Human Male,* xii. Spitzer and Whitlock's use of the term "specimen" rather than "human" or "body" is suggestive of the kind of dehumanization of the anatomical body within the VHP. I use the term "dehumanization" not in a moralistic sense, but to indicate the way in which Jernigan's body within the VHP is, even before its transformation into digital information, already conceptualized not as a human body but rather as an anatomical object.

47. Ellison, "Anatomy of a Murderer," 25.

48. Ibid., 25.

49. In a sense, as Cartwright has noted, the VHP exhibits a complete transformation of nineteenth-century criminological theory that claimed that criminal tendencies were evident in physiological anomalies or characteristics. In the case of Jernigan, it would seem this notion in the late twentieth century is informed by Cartesian dualism, where physiology and psychology are presupposed to be completely disparate, such that an ideal anatomical body can exist in combination with a deviant or abnormal psyche. Cartwright, "Cultural Anatomy," 24.

50. Michael Janover, "Nostalgias," *Critical Horizons* 1, no. 1 (2000), 113–33. Janover cites Proust's comment that "the only true paradise is always the paradise we have lost" (127.)

51. M. Ashraf Aziz and James C. McKenzie, "The Dead Can Still Teach the Living: The Status of Cadaver-Based Anatomy in the Age of Electronic Media," *Perspectives in Biology and Medicine* 1999 42, no. 3 (1999), 408–09.

52. Ibid., 409.

53. As Csordas questions, "What will be the consequences of digital dissection that is both exceedingly neat and comfortably reversible in comparison to actual dissec-

tion, in much the same way word processing allows easy deletion and substitution in comparison to writing or typing?" Csordas, "Computerized Cadavers," 187–88.

54. Spitzer and Whitlock, *Atlas of the Visible Human Male*, xix.

# SEVEN

# Endography

## *A Physician's Dream of Omniscience*

---

### CATHERINE BELLING

> ...the thought..
> Doth (like a poisonous mineral) gnaw my inwards...
> —William Shakespeare, *Othello*

> The famous old anatomist, Wolff, insists that the internal viscera are more variable than the external parts... He has even written a treatise on the choice of typical examples of the viscera for representation. A discussion on the beau-ideal of the liver, lungs, kidneys, etc. as of the human face divine, sounds strange in our ears.
> —Charles Darwin, *The Descent of Man*

> ...you can't do an autopsy because the patients are somewhere hovering between life and death. That makes it even more important that you do another kind of "opsy," a *live-opsy*, if you will.
> —Robin Cook, *Coma*

"LIVE-OPSY" IS AN UNCOMFORTABLE WORD. A terminological problem I encountered when I began writing this chapter has gradually become its subject: There is no word in English for all the bodily material contained by the skin, and no word for gaining access to that material while it is alive.

As is often the case with terminological lacunae, this one points to an epistemological problem. We do not, even with the help of biomedical science and technology, have real access to the inside of living bodies as they live. The narration of events happening inside bodies, which I will call "endography," is a physician-novelist's effort to construct and convey an impossibly omniscient interior access.

As my epigraphs show, there are plenty of words that point inward, but they do so inadequately. Iago likens the experience of envy to having poison consume his internal organs, his "inwards" (the word, corrupted, became the butchery term "innards"). Darwin describes the way in which Caspar Friedrich Wolff, the eighteenth-century German founder of embryology, thought of the visible differences between usually invisible organs in aesthetic terms, the way we tend to compare eyes or noses or mouths. The term Darwin uses is "the internal viscera." Neither "inwards" nor "viscera" is quite adequate, though, for imagining and signifying all that the skin contains, since both are limited to the internal *organs*, the functionally individuated bodies housed mostly inside the trunk, and "innards," like "entrails," is usually limited further, to the intestines or guts. What word would also include, say, the ankle joint, the brain, the fat? "Flesh," perhaps, but this, too, is inadequate to the complexity of the body's interior, particularly when that body is alive and functioning. The inside of the body is both substance and place, the stuff as well as the site where biological events continually happen, and it is also, to our experience at least, psychosomatic: material but experientially imbued with feeling. Iago feels his envy inside him, not entirely metaphorically.

Seeking access to the interior (and I suppose this is as good and as inadequate a word as any) as object rather than as site of subjective, phenomenological, embodied experience, we imagine that access either as profoundly mediated by medical imaging technology, or as dependent on the physical violation of a body that is either dead, as in autopsy, or at least anaesthetized, as in surgery. In both cases, access is short term, limited by the stasis of death or the living body's limited tolerance for exposure to the outside. We might imagine the vivisection of conscious human beings, but it is in most contexts almost unimaginable, not least because we know that consciousness under such conditions would not last long. As I shall show, to imagine the inside of the body as a narratable space is to risk displacing the embodied mind.

We all take an interest, sooner or later, in the inside of our own bodies. Most intimate yet most inaccessible, the material interior is frequently a site of great anxiety. We may wonder whether, at any moment, things could be happening inside us, invisible and as yet intangible, that may turn out to have effects that are painful, catastrophic, even lethal. This anxiety is surely one of the reasons that medical suspense fiction became so popular. The personal medical experiences of most people are inherently suspenseful, and we rely on health care professionals to help resolve that suspense by investigating and telling us about what we contain.

In this chapter I will consider a few other words that attempt to elucidate the interior: biopsy, necropsy, tomography, endoscopy. Each points to a process that has limitations. Medical access to bodily interiors is hardly complete or infallible. Until quite recently the only way a physician could examine such interiors was invasively, by exposing them physically to the surface, through surgery or postmortem dissection. What followed from this, of course, was that nonphysicians usually had no visual access at all to the body's interior as object, rather than as the subjectively sensed interior materiality that forms the phenomenological experience of embodiment. We are now in a period of unprecedented interior visibility. The body is represented and mediated by technologies like CT scans and MRIs and more widely accessible media like television shows about medicine that feature endoscopic and invasive surgery.[1] Medical technology appears to offer its practitioners and, by extension, its patients something approaching cutaneous transparency. But this access is illusory.

In the 1970s, around the time that the more complex of imaging technologies like the CT scan began to be widely available, the rise of the medical thriller implicitly offered another way to envisage the inside of the body. This access is less seemingly direct and more frankly fictive than autopsies or X-rays but, in presenting the living body's interior as its object, it bears similar marks of medical authority. In *narrating* that interior, this writing constructs an imaginary body that, in its appeal to readers' anxieties about their own bodies, may paradoxically come closer to an experiential reality than science's objectivized images, even as it frames that fictive reality as always already constructed by the discourse of biomedicine.

Two discursive genres, clinical medicine and suspense fiction, meet in the work of one physician-author to address, perhaps unintentionally, this problem of access and language. In his first thriller about health care, 1977's *Coma*, Robin Cook began to use the languages of medicine and fiction to fashion a bodily interior that was narratable while (fictionally) alive in new—and not altogether unproblematic—ways. Endography fulfills a doctor's fantasy of medical omniscience, and it can be realized only through fiction.

As I shall show, too, the problem of access is complicated by political and ethical changes in medical practice that follow in part from changes in the role of women in medicine, both as practitioners and as patients. Central to *Coma* are two female bodies. One young woman loses brain function during routine gynecological surgery; the other uses her medical knowledge to discover the reason for this coma even while her own body is an uneasy object of surveillance. The last part of my chapter considers "gynopsy," access to the interior of female bodies, as a particular, and particularly problematic, instance of Cook's efforts at medical knowledge and power.

Before turning to *Coma*, I use a passage from one of Cook's later novels, where the technique is more established, to illustrate what I mean by endography. This is the prologue of a 1988 thriller, *Mortal Fear*:

> October 11, Wednesday P.M.
>
> The sudden appearance of the foreign proteins was the molecular equivalent of the Black Plague. It was a death sentence with no chance of reprieve, and Cedric Harring had no idea of the drama about to happen inside him.
>
> In sharp contrast, the individual cells of Cedric Harring's body knew exactly what disastrous consequences awaited them. The mysterious new proteins that swept into their midst and through their membranes were overwhelming, and the small amounts of enzymes capable of dealing with the newcomers were totally inadequate. Within Cedric's pituitary gland, the deadly new proteins were able to bind themselves to the repressors that covered the genes for the death hormone. From that moment, the fatal genes exposed, the outcome was inevitable. The death hormone began to be synthesized in unprecedented amounts. Entering the bloodstream, the hormone coursed out into Cedric's body. No cell was immune. The end was only a matter of time. Cedric Harring was about to disintegrate into his stellar elements.[2]

What is this story? "Foreign proteins" appear, marking the beginning of a "drama" taking place inside a person. We, the readers, do not know at once where they appear, but we know more than the person in whose body this is happening. What do we see as we read? How do we imagine the "appearance" of foreign proteins? What do we think they look like? How do we envisage their arrival on a narrative scene?

Cook helps with a metaphor. First he sets a scale. The story he is telling is happening at the molecular level, a scale to which we have access only through biochemical modeling or through the finest and hence most alienating microscopy. Then he establishes an analogy on a far larger scale. The appearance of the proteins inside this single body is like the onset of a notoriously lethal epidemic in a human population. He then draws the two scales together at the level of the individual, the patient himself, given the specificity of a name, Cedric Harring. The narrative now has its setting as well as its scale: inside the particular body of Harring, at a particular time. "October 11, Wednesday P.M." reminds us that the process narrated is not a general, repeatable one, but rather a particular and situated sequence of events. Harring is already doomed but, crucially, is unaware of it; he "has no idea of the drama about to happen inside him." Happily oblivious, he is not the subject of this narrative. His oblivion, however, is designed to lead the reader to wonder what drama might be unfolding unfelt inside his or her own body at the moment of reading. The medical thriller is always finally about the bodily anxieties of its reader.

Cook endows subjectivity not on the human character but on "the individual cells of . . . Cedric Harring's body," who "know" what is going to happen next. They become the protagonists of this narrative, the first victims of the deadly proteins. To follow the plot, we do not need to know anything much about biochemistry or anatomy. Instead, Cook gives us enough information to make us trust that *he* does. There are membranes and enzymes, repressors, the pituitary gland and genes, and the synthesis of a death hormone. We can imagine a cascade of physiological processes even if we do not understand the mechanisms implied. We imagine the hormone spreading inside Cedric and we anticipate his death, even though we know nothing about him as a character in a novel. For now, he is merely the setting.

The interior narrative does more than simply present events from a tantalizingly unusual perspective, one that is "graphic," both in its bodily subject matter and its clinical detail. It also plays on a fundamental anxiety about the body's interior—that it is the site of horror stories we don't (yet) know about. Cook's narrator is, strictly, an impersonal, omniscient, apparently unsituated narrator, and yet he is also marked by his vocabulary and expertise as a physician, as Dr. Cook himself, only this Dr. Cook is endowed with access to objects and events normally inaccessible to human consciousness. Even the finest medical testing modalities would not be able to detect the initial "appearance of foreign proteins," not least because, in the absence of awareness from the patient, there would be no reason to test for them.

The novel's first chapter opens with a rapid shift to a more conventional perspective, the point of view of a human character: "The pain was like a white-hot knife starting somewhere in his chest and quickly radiating upward in blinding paroxysms to paralyze his jaw and left arm. Instantly Cedric felt the terror of the mortal fear of death" (13). With the condition's first symptom—pain—the narration shifts to a subject that is psyche instead of soma. We are more accustomed to omniscient narrators giving us access to minds than to bodies, after all. At the moment the somatic plot intersects with Harring's consciousness, he becomes subject and protagonist of the horror story that began, unnoticed, inside him.

The events of the prologue lead quickly to the death of Cedric Harring: "Darkness descended like a lead blanket" (18). We are, however, given one more glimpse inside his body. The physician performing the autopsy notes that "Cedric's heart had burst open inside his chest" (19). This is a far more conventional account of the body's interior. Its subject is human, the pathologist, and his access is based on physically opening up the body and looking at what is no longer concealed inside. This narration of the body is in the pluperfect tense. At the moment of observation, the important events have always already happened, the heart "had burst." Autopsy produces a retrospective and reconstructed narrative about the body. It is not endography; it is not rooted in "live-opsy."

The rest of this chapter focuses on what was arguably the first work in the genre of medical thrillers by physicians.[3] Robin Cook's novels (twenty-seven of them by 2007) are consistently successful sellers, despite the occasional recognition by even his loyal fans that the characters who act out his plots of health care paranoia tend to be stock cutouts speaking cardboard dialogue.[4] Yet in *Coma*, his first suspense novel, published in 1977 and the following year made into a successful film by his medical school classmate and fellow writer of bestsellers, Michael Crichton, Cook begins to establish the body's living interior as the site where doctors can tell gripping stories.[5] In the context of the popular suspense novel and the conventions of genre fiction, what emerges is a curious new body, one where medical discourse overshadows the typical fictional techniques for producing psychological "depth,"—where, one might say, two-dimensional characters are endowed with three-dimensional bodies. That such writing should arise at a time when anxieties about health care were emerging powerfully into public awareness should come as no surprise.

As I shall show, it is apt that Cook's narration of living interiors should emerge in the context of a mystery plot concerning coma patients, the uncovering of a hospital-managed conspiracy to induce coma in healthy patients in order to remove their organs and sell them for transplantation. The comatose are particularly resistant to corporeal investigation. Because alive, they may not be physically opened to scrutiny, and because unconscious, they are incapable of providing any of the usual behavioral and verbal information on which most diagnosis is based. Instead, as the protagonist of *Coma*, medical student Susan Wheeler, says to surgical resident Mark Bellows, a new kind of examination is needed, since "in coma cases you can't do an autopsy because the patients are somewhere hovering between life and death."[6] She has to coin a word for the access that she seeks.

But does medicine really lack the word she needs? Why does Cook have her say "live-opsy," replacing the Greek "bios" with the English "live" rather than using as an antonym for autopsy the perfectly serviceable "*biopsy*"? A medical biopsy involves removing a tiny sample of tissue from a

living body and examining it outside that body. Such an examination usually provides information only about the sample removed and the tissue it
was taken from, typically a tumor thereby found to be either malignant or
benign. While deductions about the entire body are of course made from
biopsy, what is seen is just a fragment of tissue. Susan means something
more substantial, a way of looking that will provide access on the scale
beyond even that provided by autopsy, access to everything going on inside
a living body.

Medicine can approximate such access in four ways: by postmortem
dissection if the life, and thus the plot to be investigated, has already
ended; by exploratory surgery such as laparotomy which, like autopsy,
opens the body's interior to the surface; by endoscopy, where instruments
are inserted in the body to illuminate, and at times operate on, parts of the
living interior either through existing passages, as in bronchoscopy or
colonoscopy, or through small artificial orifices as in laparoscopy, where a
hole is often punched in the navel; and by means of virtual access via imaging technologies. In *Coma*, Cook presents all these as possibilities, implicitly inviting readers to imagine themselves as either the investigator or the
examined body in each instance. But none, finally, can provide the kind of
real-time and long-term access that medical suspense relies on and craves.
Too invasive or too mediated or too limited in scope, these modes of
seeing into the body function, in Cook's writing and in our cultural narratives about medicine, to provoke the desire for a more complete way of
knowing the body, a kind of platonic endoscopy in which we inhabit our
own bodies, knowingly, at a material and biological level, at the levels of
the organ or the cell, as well as at the phenomenological level of the
embodied person.

I begin by examining his use in the novel of what we'd call, depending
on our choice of emphasis, autopsy or necropsy or, to follow Susan's ety-
mology, "dead-opsy": looking inside the corpse.

## NECROPSY

> What does it mean to cut open and look into the secret
> recesses of a *dead person*?
>
> —Elizabeth Klaver, *Sites of Autopsy*

The plot of *Coma* is relatively simple. A medical student on her
surgery rotation observes that things seem to go wrong in an unusual
number of minor surgeries, leaving patients comatose. She enthusiastically
embarks on an investigation, against the advice of her physician-supervi-
sors and the resident, Mark Bellows, who becomes her lover. She persists,

and uncovers a plot to keep the coma patients in a chronic care facility, where they are suspended by wires and sustained by computers, to incubate their own organs until needed for harvesting and sale. The horror of this vision, a hundred live coma patients in one room, hanging from wires screwed into their bones—their "heads were supported by...wires from the ceiling which were attached to screw eyes in the patients' skulls" (267)—reminds Susan of an encounter earlier in her medical training. She "recalled the upsetting image of the cadavers hung in the freezer" in the Gross Anatomy laboratory (267).

The cadaver used for medical school dissection is a body whose interior is of interest for its generalizability rather than its specifics. It is doubly dead, perhaps, since the student takes it apart not to learn anything about the inside of this body—anatomy dissection is not autopsy—but to learn about the structure of all bodies, or more precisely of a generic Body as object of medicine. The cadaver is, for Susan, entirely immune to "live-opsy." Hung up in a way that will be echoed by the comatose bodies—"After embalming, they were hung up with tongs hooked into the external ear canals. The tongs were connected to roller bearings on tracks in ceiling..." (243)—the cadavers' real function is as horror props. Susan is chased by a "hitman" employed by the conspirators to stop her investigation. She escapes into the empty anatomy lab, and he follows her, where he is shocked: "The head was dissected free of skin, the teeth and the eyes were bared.... The front of the chest was gone.... The organs, which had been removed, were piled back into the open body haphazardly" (243–44). This open body with its unpacked contents has no interior. Its purpose is to thwart the hitman, for Susan as a medical student is hardened to the appearance of the dead in ways that the assassin is not. She escapes by trapping him under a pile of bodies in the refrigerated storage room.

Cook also introduces actual autopsy into *Coma*. It functions as the antithesis of the access Susan needs. She visits the pathology lab in search of a patient who died in the hospital of causes she suspects may be related to her coma cases. As Susan watches, a resident reaches "into the tangle of organs with his left hand, grasping the liver.... The liver made a sloshing sound as it oozed onto the scale" (135). She learns nothing, but Cook again presents a dead body as disorganized, a "tangle." He focuses not on the knowledge gained from opening it but on the effect that imagining the opened body might have on a reader—a 1977 reader, a great deal less familiar with images of medically violated bodies than we are.[7]

There is, however, a second autopsy scene in *Coma*. Snooping about the Jefferson Institute, where the coma patients are kept, Susan observes what appears to be a postmortem examination. The body is naked and opened, and its internal organs are being removed. The words of the doctors, though, make her realize that this is a parody of autopsy: "'So much for the lungs. How much should we say the heart weighed?' said one of the voices. 'Your turn to guess,' laughed the other" (274). The body is one of the coma patients. His organs are being harvested. He is probably still alive or, rather, dying. The doctors are inventing autopsy results, presumably for the official medical record, and for the patient's family, who will not know about the organ harvest. The doctors also discuss how much money each organ will fetch on the black market. This "live-opsy" seeks profit, not knowledge.

In the next room, Susan finds the corollary of this nontherapeutic—or involuntarily altruistic—surgery: a room where the harvested organs are kept alive (in a rather more spectacular state than is usually the case with donor organs). She sees "two Plexiglass structures [that]...resembled fish tanks....The first contained a human heart, suspended in a fluid. It was quivering but not beating. The other contained a human kidney, also suspended in a fluid" (278). The patient may be dead, but the organs are not. Instead of autopsy, Cook shows us a different corollary for access to the interior: internal organs, living and functioning in full view outside the body. Here, organs continue to live like independent creatures—like fish—in transparent containers designed, unlike the body, to facilitate visual access to their contents.

As Elizabeth Klaver shows in her work on autopsy, to look inside a dead person is to become the subject to its object, to undo the secrecy of its interior recesses by uncovering them, violently, with a scalpel. But as she also shows, this apparently simple and inevitable paradigm of expert examiner and inanimate examinee is complicated both by the constructedness of the dichotomy and by another terminological problem: In the language of biomedical science—as in the term "research on human subjects," for instance—"subject" means "object."[8] When the embodied, conscious Subject$_1$ looks inside the body of Subject2, the gaze is always reflected and deflected in ways that make autopsy the seeing *of* oneself as well as a seeing *for* oneself. And when Subject$_2$ is still alive, and the cutting is with the eyes rather than the scalpel, the question of subjectivity becomes even more troubled.

Robin Cook's medical heroine learns that anatomy cadavers and post-mortem dissection will not help solve the problem of "live-opsy." The living organs Susan is able to see are premised on the death of the body that had contained them. We move then to another form of access to the interior: tomography. The word means, literally, "slice-writing." One may consider it a form of virtual vivisection.

## TOMOGRAPHY

> CAT fever is a new disease entity that has a broad clinical spectrum. The predominant symptom appears as a feverish impulse to own, operate, exploit, or write about what has been known as Computerized Axial Tomography (CAT).
>
> —*New England Journal of Medicine*, 1976

Around the time Robin Cook was writing *Coma*, computed axial tomography, or the CT scan, as it is now more commonly named, was coming to be popularly recognized as a breakthrough in medical access to the body's interior. In the CT scan, multiple cross-section X-ray images of the body are synthesized to reconstruct a three-dimensional representation that does not differentiate between inside and outside. In October and November 1975 the *New York Times* published several stories about the new technology, one headline announcing a "New View of the Body."[9] Even as it was introduced to the public as an uninvasive way to see inside the body, however, the rhetoric of cutting—slicing—informed popular descriptions of its technique. The October 1975 *Times* story describes a patient "stretched out in what looked like a guillotine about to slice through his abdomen," but adds that, "rather than a knife, this 'guillotine' would use X-rays."[10] Another article describes the scan's "bloodless incision, displaying in cross-section any part of the body."[11] Tomography as slice-writing was dissection without pain, without requiring the death or anesthetization of its "subject."

Yet despite the contagious interest in these new imaging technologies, they play a relatively small part in Cook's novel. We are given regular X-ray access—in a teaching conference on care of the comatose, the "focal point" is the "projected image of a Kodachrome of a human lung" (62–63)—but other imaging technologies are mentioned only to be rejected. For instance, a neurology resident's consult report on one of the coma patients states the following:

> Pneumoencephalography [a painful and now seldom-used method of examining the brain by temporarily replacing the cerebrospinal fluid in the skull with air and then X-raying it] and/or a CAT scan may be of help but I believe it would be of academic interest only and would not provide any additional information for diagnosis in this difficult case. (103)

It seems odd that in a "difficult case" a technology so likely to assist, if only in ruling out bleeding as a cause, should be of "academic interest only." The term suggests that such scrutiny would perhaps satisfy curiosity about the state of the patient's brain—but not answer questions about causation.

Yet a follow-up note on the next page of the chart by the same neurologist diagnoses "brain death," as a result of hypoxia, lack of oxygen, and suggests that its probable cause was "some sort of cerebral vascular accident perhaps due to a transient blood clot, platelet clot, fibrin clot or other embolus" (104). The note concludes that "Cerebral angiography, pneumoencephalography, and a CAT scan can be done, but it is the combined opinion that the results would be normal" (104). While the actual cause of the coma, carbon monoxide inhalation, would not show up on a CAT scan, other possible causes, such as an intracranial bleed, would, and these would normally need to be ruled out.

For some reason, then, Cook chooses not to include these "new views of the body" in the novel. One of the problems of imaging technology, from the thriller-writer's point of view, is its very bloodlessness. Unlike autopsy there are no actual organs to be described as materially present to the senses. The viewing subject of this technology sees clearly mediated and stylized reconstructions of the interior. No matter how valid the information they provide, such images do not provide direct access to the interior itself.

Imaging technology is also limited in its ability to capture change over time. Just as autopsy examines a body where the story is no longer taking place, the pathologist reconstructing events that have already happened from an unmoving, dead interior, so imaging technology takes the dynamic living body and reduces it to a snapshot, the capture of one moment in its interior life. A *Times* article describes "a prototype unit that may one day be incorporated into a device that scans in one one-hundredth of a second—fast enough to 'stop' the motion of a beating heart."[12] It still has to stop the heart, rather than capturing the motion itself.

The problem of learning about the dynamic living body with the technologies of stasis is raised explicitly by Cook in *Coma*. A resident describes the difficulty of tracking a comatose patient's internal condition: "What we need to check is the exact amount of fluid the patient has put out versus the exact amount that has been given. Of course this is static data and we are more interested in the dynamic state. But we can get a pretty good idea" (42). In the Jefferson Institute, where the technology constitutes "modern medicine taken to the nth degree" (268), knowledge about interiors is also dependent on deduction from the measurement of physiological values and output, and its new technologies, invented by Cook for the novel and clearly admired by him despite their scandalously unethical context, are better at capturing change than existing methods:

> …weight, blood gases, fluid balance, blood pressure, body temperature…are being constantly scanned and compared to standards by the

computer.... It is far better than conventional care. A doctor tends to concern himself with isolated variables and in a static fashion. The computer is
able to sample over time, hence it treats dynamically. But more important
still is that the computer correlates all the variables at any given moment.
It's much more like the body's own regulatory mechanisms. (268)

This physiological dynamism characterizes living bodies, but is almost
always put on hold or concealed when the body is under scrutiny. Even
when the body can be looked into, its interior cannot be *watched*.

In her study of the parallel developments of cinema and medical imaging in the twentieth century, Lisa Cartwright points out that film could
capture the temporality of the living body in a way that still photography—
and postmortem dissection—could not.[13] Medicine's interest in anatomy,
autopsy, and imaging technology lies predominantly not in a desire to
learn about the structure or condition of corpses or the state of a body at
the moment it is scanned. All these approaches are the best we have for
approximating access to the dynamic state of the living body, the body
that, no matter its condition at the moment of attention, is always in
process—a process that is always a movement toward death. To capture this
process, something other than the retrospect of the autopsy or the immedi-
acy of the scan is needed. The discourse that comes closest, whether purely
verbal, or visual like cinema, is narrative. In *Mortal Fear*, we saw how Cook
narrated the onset of a disease crisis happening inside the body of an oblivious not-yet-patient. There is one more form of access to the living body's
interior that seems likely to provide something like the possibility of narrative: the therapeutic vivisection we call surgery.

## SURGERY

> The knife was then inserted into the joint and for a few
> moments Dr. Spallek rooted around blindly, his face
> upturned toward the ceiling. He was cutting by feel
> alone. There was a faint grinding sound, then a snap.
>
> — *Coma*

The surgery described above—a meniscectomy, the removal of a piece
of damaged cartilage from the knee joint—would now usually be done by
sight as well as feel. Arthroscopy allows a camera to enter the joint and
guide the surgeon who watches the procedure on a television monitor. In
1977, this was not an option. The patient having the knee surgery here is
the same one Susan later sees having his organs harvested at the
Jefferson Institute.

The central site of anxiety in *Coma* is the operating room. It is here that patients admitted for minor surgery are rendered comatose by receiving carbon monoxide rather than oxygen during anaesthesia. But this is special. The operating room is also, of course, where patients' bodies are routinely cut open and exposed. It is revealing, then, that even in his accounts of surgery in the novel, Cook does not provide close descriptions of a body opened to access.

Before discussing Cook's descriptions of surgery, I want to consider briefly the meaning of the "graphic" in writing about the body. The *OED*'s primary definition captures the visuality of the term: "Producing by words the effect of a picture; vividly descriptive, life-like."[14] Writing is used to *draw* a detailed visual image for the reader. A recent addition to the dictionary narrows this definition to the bodily: "Providing or conveying full, unexpurgated detail; expressly stated or represented; explicit, esp. in the depiction of sex or violence"—that is, in the depiction of actions involving the body, especially those parts of the body not routinely available to view, exposed to description only because of sexual activity or violation of the body's surface. Or by medical intervention.

A critic describing Robin Cook's account of surgery uses the term as follows: "The clinical details ... are presented with graphic realism (down to the snapping sound of the latex gloves Dr. Foley puts on) and Cook thus establishes the aura of authenticity that his depiction of medical procedures inevitably evokes."[15] It is perhaps surprising that the sound of gloves should be considered evidence of Cook's authoritative medical and surgical experience. But the paradox in the accounts of surgery in *Coma* is that the most "graphic" access the reader is given to the inside of bodies does not involve the patient. Despite the literally opened body present in the room, Cook's real interest, as I have suggested, is in the interiors of people who are not cadavers, or surgical patients, or subject to imaging technologies, but rather resemble the probable reader: alive, awake, and functioning as dynamic setting to physiological processes that could be narrated, continually, if one could only apprehend them. Cook's narration offers this illusory, medicine-dependent, and anxiogenic grasp, and he uses surgery as a trigger for the far more medically *graphic*, but neither sexual nor necessarily violent, narration I call "endography." The interiority that interests Cook is invisible to the others in the room, even the surgeons. It is available only to his medically omniscient narrator and to the reader.

Another scene in *Coma* exemplifies this. The medical students on their surgical rotation, including Susan, attend their first surgery, a gall bladder removal. Cook begins to describe the procedure from the point of view of the students—for them, it "was like watching an execution. Their

minds tried to prepare themselves for the image that was going to be immi-
nently transmitted to their brains" (37)—already, somatic brains are separated from minds that seem like vulnerable subjects in a medicalized
environment. The students watch the opening incision:

> Johnston [the surgeon] held the scalpel about two inches above the pale
> skin.... [The anesthesiologist] looked up at Johnston and gave an imper-
> ceptible nod, tripping the poised guillotine. The scalpel dived deep into
> the tissues, and then with a smooth soundless slice, slid down the skin at
> an angle of approximately 45 degrees. The wound fell open and little jets
> of pulsating arterial blood sprayed the area, then ebbed and died. (37)

The patient's body is cut open but we do not see what those present see
when the wound falls open. Instead, Cook shifts now to his omniscient
narrator—the one who watches what happens inside living bodies where no
one can see:

> Meanwhile curious phenomena occurred in [medical student] George
> Niles's brain. The image of the knife plunging into the skin of the patient
> was displayed instantly in his occipital cortex. Association fibers picked
> up the message and transported the information to his parietal lobe,
> where it was associated. The association spread so rapidly and so widely
> that it activated an area of his hypothalamus, causing widespread dilation
> of the blood vessels in his muscles. The blood literally drained from his
> brain to fill all the dilated vessels, causing George Niles to lose conscious-
> ness. In a dead faint he fell straight backwards. (37)

The observing subject becomes object of physiological observation. Even
before he loses consciousness, the mind of George Niles is of far less interest in this text than his brain and his vascular system. This kind of graphic
writing is about establishing authority—the writer reminds the reader that
he is a doctor and understands how these things work and that, therefore,
he should be trusted when he describes more complex and perhaps troubling medical events. Cook is saying that he understands how fainting
works. He is implying more, though, too: Just as in his account of "foreign
proteins" leading to Cedric Harring's death, Cook names his character and
contextualizes his description. He is not providing a general account—"this
is what happens when a person faints"—but the far more unusual narrative
of a particular interior event—"this is what happened inside George Niles
when he fainted in the operating room on the first day of his surgery rotation." Only George Niles's creator—Robin Cook, MD, or the narrator he
has invented—could tell us this.

There are other instances of this interior narration in *Coma*, many of them on the periphery of surgery, as if the vivisection somehow illuminates the bodies around the table. An anaesthesist responds physically to a shift in one patient's blood pressure: "something was keying-off his sixth sense, activating his adrenals and pushing up his own heart rate. He watched the breathing bag" (10). This might almost work from the point of view of the character; as a physician, he may almost apprehend his own anxiety reaction in terms of adrenalin rushes and palpitations. Another instance, however, produces a stranger mix of the clinical and the experiential: "Perspiration coalesced on Dr. Goodman's forehead and dripped off the bridge of his nose onto the anesthesia record. His own heart rate was over one hundred per minute" (75-76). The subject registering Dr. Goodman's heart rate is very unlikely to be the character himself, and no one else is taking his pulse. The perspective here is that of a narrator who is both a physician and omniscient. He has equal access to the subjective mental interiority of the characters and to the physical interior that is only partially accessible to the subject himself, even as it is an object entirely available to Cook's narrator.

The anesthetized surgical patient seems to work as a fulcrum around which Cook's medically graphic but nonviolent narration of living interiors turns. Similarly, the novel's comatose patients, suspended from wires in the Jefferson Institute, have a kind of antinarrative function, their bodies as inaccessible as their minds. Set against these mindless bodies is one more kind of body, qualitatively different from the others, not because of the accessibility of its interior but because its female exterior is desirable enough to deflect—or divert—the penetrating medical eye. Yet the mind inhabiting this particular body is disconcertingly incisive itself, for it is a mind, like Cook's, trained in medicine. This psychosomatic combination threatens at times to confound Cook's careful merging of his own dual identities as thriller-writer and medical man.

The final section of this chapter considers the problem of the living female body: Whether comatose or conscious, its status illuminates the contradictions in medicine's efforts to observe the interior workings of bodies that are alive. Susan Wheeler, in the role of female physician (though she has not yet achieved that status), desires impossible knowledge of bodies—"live-opsy." Her desire and her very different desirability complicate Cook's own dream of medical omniscience (and, as we shall see, omnipotence). Even though she is Cook's creation, Susan's mind threatens the dual body—attractive outside and accessible within—that he is trying to write.

## GYNOPSY

> The dilation of the cervix went without a hitch. Nancy
> had a normally antero-flexed uterus, and the curve on
> the dilators was a perfect match. A few blood clots were
> sucked from the vaginal vault.
>
> —*Coma*

The first coma patient described in the novel is Nancy Greenly, a young woman admitted for a D&C to treat irregular menses. The book's prologue is an account of her gynecological surgery. It begins: "Nancy Greenly lay on the operating table on her back, staring up at the large...lights in operating room No. 8, trying to be calm" (1). Soon Nancy is anesthetized, given carbon monoxide instead of oxygen, and rendered comatose. The subject position that opens the novel, that of the female patient, is rapidly obliterated as Nancy becomes one of the inanimate living bodies that resist access. Her point of view is replaced by the perspectives of the surgical team, first Dr. Majors, the surgeon, who dilates Nancy's cervix and scrapes her endometrium—observing that her ovaries "felt like little smooth, normal plums" (9)—and then by the anesthetist who realizes that something has gone wrong when her blood pressure drops and the pupils of her eyes become fixed and dilated.

Cook's choice of a young female patient as the novel's first coma case is significant in that it allows him to introduce the interior of the female body early on in the novel both as site of sexual anxiety and as a place where the medical can interact with the sexualized in providing, as in his description of the dilation and curettage of Nancy Greenly's cervix and uterus, a close but clinical look at a woman's reproductive organs. Before being anesthetized, Nancy reflects on her condition—irregular menses—and its treatment, and Cook establishes a contradiction between the outward and the interior: "She was a delicately angular and attractive girl with an aristocratic appearance. About her person she was fastidious.....So the continued bleeding made her feel messy, unattractive, out of control" (2-3). Nancy has a romantic weekend planned and the bleeding will make her sexually unavailable. The treatment, however, only adds to her shame: "She was grateful, because it [surgery] was going to help her...; she was furious because she felt so exposed, literally and figuratively" (6). The pelvic exam is a traumatic experience: "A flimsy curtain, which was constantly being whisked back and forth, was the sole barrier between the throng in the emergency room and Nancy's flayed self-respect" (3). Surgeon and reader share access to Nancy's reproductive organs. We see blood in her vaginal vault and, like Caspar Wolff, Darwin's embryologist, medicine lets us make judgments about internal organs: Nancy's uterus is a

"perfect match" for the surgeon's tools. At the same time, Cook's narrator
has access to Nancy's brain as she is anesthetized—"the Phenergan and
Demerol...were beginning to exert their effects somewhere within the
depths of her cerebrum" (4). The "effects" may be accessible to Nancy herself, but the drugs and their action can be known only by the physician-
narrator who can read both her mind and her brain.

Once Nancy is comatose, a new female protagonist is introduced.
Susan Wheeler, the medical student, is exactly the same age as Nancy and,
encountering her for the first time only after the disastrous surgery, she
identifies with her on several levels. "Without the aid of extensive clinical
experience, Susan was instantly lost in the human element. The age and
sex similarity struck too close to home for her to avoid the identification"
(43). Before learning of the conspiracy, Susan attributes Nancy's coma to
the interaction between medicine and her particularly female body:
"Nancy Greenly, as immobile as a statue, a casualty of medicine, a victim
of technology. Susan wondered about her life, her loves. Everything was
gone, all because of a simple menstrual irregularity, a routine D&C" (61).
Imagining herself in Nancy's place is what begins Susan's efforts to discover the cause of the coma cases.

But Susan is not a disembodied medical mind seeking answers to a
diagnostic problem. As a popular novelist, Cook makes bodies for his
female characters that are designed largely as objects of his (and, presumably, his imagined readers') desire. Resident Mark Bellows looks, unclini-
cally, at Susan: "As she [stood up], her blouse fell away from her chest..."
(115). He admires "her splendid breasts, barely contained by a flimsy bra,
their skin of a smoothness Bellows imagined to be like velvet" (116). Finally
she sits down again, hiding her chest and "relieving the stress on Bellows's
hypothalamus" (116). The narrator remains clinical even when the surgical
resident is not.

The frank objectification of Susan's body, typical as it may have been
in many 1970s genre novels, is at odds with her subject position as medical
investigator of other bodies. It also, however, reflects a conflict experienced
at the time by women becoming physicians. It is as if being embodied as a
woman upset the subject-object balance needed for clinical observation.
Susan experiences the performativity of the doctor role as in conflict with
her body: "She felt transparent as if she were an actress playing the role of
a doctor. She had on the white coat and the scene was melodramatic and
appropriate. Yet on the inside she just didn't feel like the part, and there
was the thought that she would be exposed at any moment as a charlatan"
(49). The doctor's white coat is a costume marking a very particular part of
the doctor role; it is the lab coat, symbol of scientific objectivity, eliding
the physician's body into an ideal position of detached observational

omniscience—a position rather like that of Cook's endographic narrator. Susan fears that, inside the coat, she has the wrong body.

She considers the implications of medicine for her identity, referring again to the problem that links her with the comatose Nancy Greenly: "She felt female and her monthly menstrual flow emphasized its reality. But was she a woman?" (60). One wonders whether any woman has ever relied on menstruation as evidence of her sex, but of course what Susan thinks is not the thinking of a woman, but of the male doctor who writes her mind as well as her body. Cook's intentions are clearly, at one level, to try to support the acceptance of women into medicine as equal professionals to men, and to address the difficulties this may pose for female doctors. In an author's note at the end of *Coma*, he describes some of the bioethical realities he had hoped to alert readers to (problems of access to donor organs, for instance), and he concludes with a "final word about women in medicine: I must admit," he writes, "that the research I did on the subject...caused me to alter my opinions. I now have a heightened regard for female physicians and female medical students. I recognize that their training experiences are much more difficult and stressful than those of their male counterparts" (308).

At the same time, Susan's body remains stubbornly that of the female heroine of a genre novel: the object of visual desire. As a student, Susan finds this inconvenient:

> Having entered a profession dominated by males, in which essentially all the professors and instructors were males, Susan Wheeler could not skip a class without being missed. Despite the fact that Susan looked on her mentors in a neutral sexless way as her professional superiors, they did not return the view in kind. The fact of the matter was that Susan Wheeler was a very attractive twenty-three year old female. (12)

Cook has the resident Mark Bellows address the problem surprisingly directly. As we have seen, he desires Susan, but he fears becoming involved with her, not for professional reasons but for epistemological ones. He worries that her mind will not match what he wants from her body: "Bellows did not reduce his own sexual urges and fantasies to anatomical and physiological realities, but what about Susan?" (159). This is of course exactly the kind of reductiveness Cook employs in describing Bellows's desire as "stress on his hypothalamus" (116), but in a woman, Bellows fears, so incisive an understanding of what happens inside the body would be hazardous indeed:

> She looked so normal with her smile, her soft skin, the hint of her breast gently rising with her breathing. But she had studied the parasympathetic

reflexes, and the endocrine alterations that make sex possible, even enjoy-able. Maybe she had studied too much, too much of the wrong thing. Maybe even if the occasion was auspicious, Bellows would find his penis limp, impotent. (159)

Female medical knowledge demystifies sex, reducing it to biomedicine and threatening to render the male—in particular, the male MD—impotent. Cook's generic and so-1970s-masculine physician-narrator has the author-ity to narrate the body's interior. Susan's ability to imagine change and process—narrative—inside the body makes her, paradoxically and for Cook perhaps unintentionally, a threat to that authority. Her knowledge threat-ens to emasculate Mark Bellows. It also threatens and finally overthrows the power of the medical establishment that is running the murderous organ harvest program, for this is a conspiracy of the establishment. At its head is the Boston Memorial Hospital's Chief of Surgery.

At the end of the novel, Susan's identification with Nancy comes full circle. We return to the operating room, but now Susan is the patient. Having solved the coma mystery, she foolishly tells the chief of surgery what she has learned. To keep her from telling, he drugs her and has her rushed to the OR for an unneeded emergency appendectomy, planning to ensure that she will be the next coma victim. Our last access to Susan as protagonist is as she loses consciousness: "An anesthesia mask dropped over her face. . . . She saw someone thrust a syringe into the I.V. line" (303).

Mark Bellows, the resident, realizes what is happening and is able to interrupt the surgery, though not before Susan has had her abdomen opened and her appendix removed. The appendix is an inessential organ, but nonetheless an echo remains of the earlier organ harvest. The novel ends with Susan still unconscious. She has received at least some carbon monoxide. Cook does not reveal—or decide, perhaps—whether her brain has been damaged or not. The central knowing subject of the novel, though, is completely elided from its conclusion. Susan's efforts at "live-opsy" end with her own living body opened and examined and parts of her dissected. Her mind is not part of the end of the story.

In a way, then, *Coma* might be seen as a novel about the (gendered) potency of the medical profession in the 1970s, where the rise of bioethics, with its new insistence on patient autonomy and informed consent and its roots in the human rights and women's movements, was calling into ques-tion the trusted paternalistic power, and power over knowledge, of the physician. Cook's effort to addresses contemporary issues, such as the entry of women into the medical profession, in the context of popular fic-tion illuminates the contradictions that characterize medicine's construc-tion and representation of the human body. Women's bodies, where the exterior is so conventionally objectivized, are perhaps the most noticeable site of these contradictions, but the real problem goes deeper. Medicine relies for its power on access to knowledge, but the omniscience it seeks and the omnipotence it imagines remain out of reach, particularly when that knowledge has as its object a human being who is both subject of medical investigation *and* bearer of its own embodied subject position. Throughout the many bestselling novels he has gone on to write, Cook endows his narrators with the ability to tell us fascinating stories about things happening inside living bodies. At the same time, he endows his characters with clichéd, stock outward characteristics, strained dialogue, shallow motivation.

Susan's description of the comatose patients captures a distinction that I think (perhaps unkindly) could also describe the characters in Robin Cook's novels: "The victim's upper brain is destroyed. He's a living corpse, but his organs are alive and warm and happy until they can be taken out..." (291). The interior of the living body, where we cannot go, even with all the access that medical technology can give us, is where Cook's characters are most alive. Readers willing to think of themselves as similarly medicalized can forgive the very schematic subjects inhabiting these interiors. Robin Cook the physician has found, in the endographic narrative created by Robin Cook the novelist, a way to write the body's interior that grants an omniscience of which medicine can only dream.

## NOTES

1. For a rich exploration of the implications of this mediated access, see José van Dijck, *The Transparent Body: A Cultural Analysis of Medical Imaging* (Seattle: University of Washington Press, 2005). Van Dijck questions the idea that "new imaging technologies" simply "lift the veil from the interior body" (16). I agree. While they do make knowledge about the living interior more available than ever before, the access is far from transparency (a tricky ideal in itself: for the kind of access desired a literally transparent body would of course be no use at all—a body with layers that can be rendered selectively transparent, perhaps?).

2. Robin Cook, *Mortal Fear* (New York: Putnam, 1988), 11. Hereafter cited in text. The "death hormone" Cook refers to is DECO, or Decreasing Oxygen Consumption Hormone. Normally, it is produced by the pituitary gland in increasing amounts as the organism (human or animal) gets older, and it reduces cells' efficiency at converting food into energy. This slowing of metabolic rate leads to the process of aging and, eventually, death.

3. While suspense-inducing fiction concerning medical subject matter of course preceded Cook's work—*Frankenstein* comes to mind at once, and one could go back

a great deal further, perhaps to plague in Thucydides—I argue elsewhere that the medical thriller novel, where anxiety is provoked both by illness or injury *and* by a health care-related conspiracy, is a particular product of the 1970s.

4. For example: "Robin Cook is definitely a doctor. Due to the nature of the novel I was more than prepared to have a fair amount of medical terminology and jargon thrown at me...at times it was a bit tedious and the explanations quite lengthy, but for the most part the subject matter kept me interested. However, I was surprised at how sterile and predictable the main characters were written." Erica Starks, Amazon.com reader review, *Coma*, July 16, 2005, http://www.amazon.com/exec/obidos/tg/detail/-/0451207394/qid=1121719939/sr=8-1/ref=pd_bbs_1/002-4126779-3096855?v=glance&s=books &n=507846, accessed July 18, 2005.

5. Before *Coma*, Cook published *The Year of the Intern* (New York: Harcourt Brace Jovanovich, 1972), a fictionalized account of his own first year as a resident.

6. Cook, *Coma*, 128, my emphasis.

7. A review of the film version of *Coma* reminds us of this: "*Coma* presents us with everything you always knew about but were afraid to see: autopsies, abortions, cadavers whole and sliced, and a vast assortment of gleaming inner organs.... There's a perfect queasy logic in setting a horror film in a hospital, but I wonder if [Michael Crichton, the director] and Cook, who are both doctors and thus professionally immune to anatomical squeamishness, haven't misjudged the audience's tolerance for the clinical" (David Ansen, "Horror Show," *Newsweek*, February 6, 1978, 86). As it turned out, Ansen was wrong: The film was a box office success.

8. Elizabeth Klaver, *Sites of Autopsy in Contemporary Culture* (Albany: SUNY Press, 2005). For a full discussion of the problem of the subject in autopsy see her chapter 3, "Autopsy and the Subject or, What the Dead Saw."

9. Jane E. Brody, "3-Dimensional X-Ray is Tested for New View of Body," *New York Times*, October 22, 1975, 89.

10. Brody, "3-Dimensional X-Ray," 89.

11. Stacy V. Jones, "X-Ray of Entire Body Shows Color TV Image," *New York Times*, November 29, 1975, 35.

12. Brody, "3-Dimensional X-Ray, 89.

13. "Although pathological anatomy, the area of Foucault's concern, centered its representations on a static concept of morphology and structure, physiology—the discipline for which the film motion study was a crucial technique—regarded the body in terms of its living functions and processes, and its practitioners devised methods and techniques to facilitate a temporal, dynamic vision of the body in motion." Lisa Cartwright, *Screening the Body: Tracing Medicine's Visual Culture* (Minneapolis: University of Minnesota Press, 1995), 11.

14. "Graphic." *The Oxford English Dictionary OED Online* (Oxford: Oxford University Press, 2004), http://www.oed.com.

15. Lorena Laura Stookey, *Robin Cook: A Critical Companion* (Westport: Greenwood Press, 1996), 92.

EIGHT

# Designer Vaginas

ALEXA A. PRIDDY AND JENNIFER L. CROISSANT

FROM THE AIRBRUSHED "PERFECTION" OF the pages of *Playboy* to the cosmetic surgeon's "perfection" of the flesh and blood body, the vagina is a visible cultural commodity in the United States. The elective cosmetic surgery procedures popularly referred to as "designer vaginas" construct female genitals to conform to societal ideals of femininity. This chapter explores the significance of the designer vagina in the fabrication of the female body. Here, we argue that the growing continuum of body projects and the discourses on designer vaginas, whether scholarly or in popular media, are indicative of how women's bodies are constructed and valued in U.S. culture today, a construction that is tightly bound to the perceived agency and choice of the individual seeking a designer vagina. Furthermore, we assert that U.S. discourses about female circumcision in other cultures contrast to designer vaginas in such a way that, despite the similarities of the surgeries, the conventional discourse of female circumcision serves to legitimate the designer vagina in contemporary U.S. culture. Through an exploration of the concept of constrained agency, we will further explore the current dilemma of women's agency and body projects. Every day women negotiate their status in U.S. culture, an act that exemplifies both their ability to exert agency in their lives and the constraints they face.

## DEFINING DESIGNER VAGINAS

A designer vagina, female genital cosmetic surgery, is most commonly marketed as a tool to improve genital aesthetics and sexual pleasure for

173

females. Because the designer vagina procedures are not acknowledged as official cosmetic surgeries by any medical association, nor can a surgeon be certified to perform these procedures, there are no official statistics on designer vaginas. What information that can be garnered is anecdotal accounts from patients in popular media and on doctors' Web sites. There has been no official study conducted that explores the frequency of these surgical procedures, the long-term effects, the demographic of patients, and so on. What we do know begins the sketch and is an important foundation for creating an understanding of designer vaginas and their implications for the future of women's bodies.

In popular media, the designer vagina can refer to any number of procedures, including vaginal rejuvenation, designer vaginoplasty (which includes labiaplasty), G-Spot amplification, and hymenoplasty. In addition to these procedures, skin can be removed from around the clitoris to increase sensitivity, and skin pigmentation can be made more homogenous. During the first procedure, vaginal rejuvenation, the surgeon decreases the diameter of the vagina and makes it tighter. This is sold as a treatment for women who have urinary incontinence, are aging, or have given birth and lost elasticity in their vagina. The primary motivation for this surgery is "for the enhancement of sexual gratification" for women, though their male partners also stand to benefit from this modification.[1]

A second category of vaginal surgery is designer vaginoplasty, which often refers to labiaplasty, pubic liposuction, and other aesthetic surgeries. Labiaplasty is the resculpting of the labia minora and labia majora. The surgeon can create "puffy" or "pouty" labia majora in order to fix those that appear "flattened" as a result of aging or childbirth. In addition, "saggy" or "unusually long" labia minora can be shortened or trimmed.[2] In Figure 8.1, the before and after pictures of a labiaplasty—labia minora reduction—are presented from Dr. Gary Alter's Web site, altermd.com. The labia minora in photographs A and B are much larger than in the postsurgery images of C and D. The designer vagina aesthetic values smaller female genitals, an aesthetic we will explore in more detail later.

G-Spot amplification and hymenoplasty are the final two procedures addressed in our analysis. G-Spot amplification involves injecting collagen into the front wall of the vagina, "making it puff up and become more prominent." The process takes approximately ten minutes and lasts up to four months. The result is supposed to be increased sexual satisfaction. Another procedure, hymenoplasty, is also called "hymen reconstruction." With this procedure, the surgeon will, as one patient says, "put a few stitches inside you where the hymen used to be. Then, when you have sex they tear and you bleed, just like when you're a virgin."[3] This procedure is often performed on women who must prove their virginity for marriage or

Image A. Before

Image B. Before

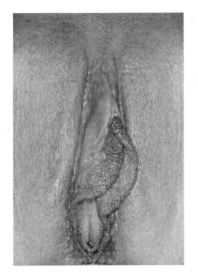

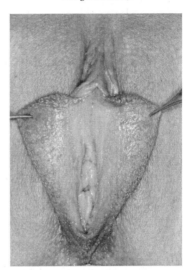

Image C. After

Image D. After

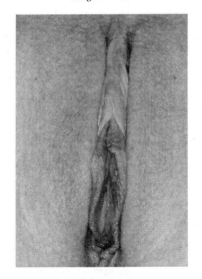

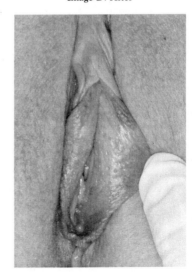

**Figure 8.1.** Designer vagina. Patient 2. 50 year old. Courtesy of Gary J. Alter, MD.

who want to provide their male partner with the "gift" of their virginity. For each of the designer vagina procedures detailed above, the cost can range from approximately $2,500 to $15,000.[4]

Although the few procedures detailed above do not represent all the possibilities of designer vagina surgery, the procedures presented here are typical of the range of procedures available to patients. These procedures are often explained in popular magazines and Web sites, which a woman seeking information about designer vaginas might be more likely to read, not the technical and medical language used by the doctors who perform designer vagina surgeries. The term *designer* vagina is representative of the popular media construction of these procedures.

Since the cost is more than just a trip to the grocery store or an expensive night out, we wonder how many women are seeking these surgeries and how they are affording them. It is difficult to answer this question with certainty. However, what we do know is that in a 2005 press release from the American Association of Plastic Surgeons, so-called fringe plastic surgery procedures, designer vaginas among them, comprised only a small fraction of the plastic surgeries performed in 2004. In fact, designer vaginal rejuvenation was performed only 793 times in 2004, which means that cosmetic surgeries such as liposuction (performed 323,605 times in 2004) and breast augmentation (performed 291,350 times in 2004) still comprise the vast majority of cosmetic and plastic surgeries performed each year in the United States.[5] Financing for designer vaginas is available for most women seeking a surgery, yet such surgeries are not covered by insurance as they are deemed cosmetic and not a medical necessity. As a result, most women will have to have a certain level of financial security to even think about purchasing or financing one of these "luxury" vaginas. Says Jane, a thirty-four-year-old woman from the Midwest who spoke about her procedure to the Detroit alternative weekly magazine *MetroTimes*, "Price was an issue for me—I financed part of this. My guess is a lot of women who do this have a lot of money. I would consider it a luxury. Not to say that I don't think it should be covered by insurance, because I think it should be."[6] Designer vaginas and other cosmetic surgeries are not accessible to most women largely because they are not covered by insurance, if a woman even has access to insurance.

According to the Web site of Dr. Matlock, owner of the Laser Vaginal Rejuvenation Institute in Los Angeles, most surgeries take approximately an hour, giving the impression that they are quick, harmless, come with few ill effects, and will instantly facilitate great sex. However, these procedures are real surgical operations, most of which are done in a hospital. The average patient waits approximately two to three months before she is healed and able to have sex without pain. The after-affects of the surgery can vary, but, as one woman reports, "the pain was excruciating. I had to wear a catheter for two days to prevent infection and I felt constantly sick. Every time I moved, my vagina and stomach would contract. Compared to childbirth, I've still never felt pain like it." Another woman says, "When I woke up...my pubic hair was congealed with blood and I felt so bruised I couldn't sit down properly for a few weeks. I kept telling myself that it would get better, that it would be all worth it."[7] Kathryn Pauly Morgan, in "Women and the Knife," believes that the use of the term "cosmetic" to describe these surgeries is misleading. In actuality, Morgan believes the term disguises the fact that they are in fact "noncosmetic" changes in that "they involve lengthy periods of pain, are permanent, and result in irreversibly alienating metamorphoses such as the appearance of youth on an aging body."[8]

In the context of our analysis, we argue that designer vaginas represent the concept of constrained agency: when the constraints imposed on a woman seeking a designer vagina—cultural constructions of beauty, idealized female sexuality, gender oppression, body image, and race, class, ethnicity, age, and ability—intersect with the agency she possesses—changing her body for herself, seeking internal and external acceptance, improving the quality of her life, self-esteem, and controlling choices over her body. Ophira Edut, editor of *Body Outlaws*, says in the Detroit *MetroTimes*, "It's a tricky subject [seeking a designer vagina]. I respect a woman's choice, and she should be the ultimate authority on her body and what to do with it. But at the same time, if a labiaplasty is what you really think it will take to make you happy, it might be time to re-examine your idea of happiness."[9]

Iris Lopez illustrates this intersection of agency and constraint in her study that problematizes the reproductive situations of Puerto Rican women in New York City. Lopez argues that women have real and valid feelings of agency but that all choices have social constraints. She states, "Presenting women as active agents of their reproductive decisions does not suggest that they are exercising free will or that they are not oppressed but that they make decisions within the limits of their constraints."[10] Like Lopez, who says, "I reformulate the binary model between submission and agency," we will similarly reformulate the binary model of cosmetic surgery—as being either a response to societal pressures *or* an act of free choice of one's body—in order to analyze designer vaginas.[11]

## HISTORICAL UNDERPINNINGS

Ideas about female genitals intersect with the construction of female sexuality. Readings of genitals have denoted hermaphoditism, homosexuality, transexuality, and/or the categorization of a body as male or female. In the introduction of Alice Domurat Dreger's *Hermaphrodites and the Medical Invention of Sex*, Dreger argues, "Clitorises and penises, for instance, come in a wide range of shapes and sizes even in people labeled 'normal' in terms of their sex."[12] In present-day representations of genitalia there appears the same need for differentiation that categorizes genitals as either male or female. This is what Judith Butler refers to as "anatomical essentialism," where the body denotes the person.[13] In contemporary U.S. culture, we argue, designer vaginas function to normalize female genitals, producing sameness among female sexual organs and distinction between male and female sexual organs.

Just as historical representations of what was considered "deviant" sexuality inform the present-day discourse of designer vaginas, so too does the U.S. feminist self-help health movement that took place in the 1970s and into the early 1980s. This movement's emphasis on understanding one's own body, taking control of it, and using technology to enhance it is similar to earlier precursors of the designer vagina and therefore itself becomes one of many precursors to the development of designer vagina procedures. The feminist self-help health movement argued that bodies are heterogeneous but made homogenous by medical texts and the "medical men" of which Dreger speaks. "Medical men" determined anatomy texts and what constituted an acceptable body in the eyes of Western medicine. However, self-help activists of the 1970s advocated for individual control of bodies. Through education women could understand their genitals, reproductive organs, and their function and not view them as the "black hole" of the body, the part of the body that was unknown to them. As Lisa Jean Moore and Adele Clarke note, many self-helpers took the inequalities they saw between the representations of female and male bodies in the anatomy texts and reinvented female representations in their own texts in an effort to amend the relative absence of female bodies. The anatomy texts would often label only the reproductive organs and not the sexual organs of the female body, like the clitoris. Therefore, self-helpers took it upon themselves to represent the female genitals as intricate sexual organs equipped with various dimensions and parts. The clitoris represented in self-help health books had three parts—the clitoral hood, the clitoral shaft, and the clitoral glans—and sometimes more, while medical texts labeled only the clitoris or left it out all together. The self-help movement's emphasis on body control constructed genital representations that challenged and contrasted with traditional anatomy texts.

This empowerment language of the self-help health movement of the 1970s is now being appropriated by some surgeons to sell the designer vaginas procedures. One surgeon states that, "Our Mission is to empower woman, with knowledge, choice and alternatives."[14] On one page of this surgeon's Web site—the Laser Vaginal Rejuvenation Institute of Los Angeles—titled "Designer Laser Vaginoplasty," the procedures that are described under this heading are explained with the aid of a diagram. This diagram exemplifies the surgeon's emphasis on empowerment by labeling multiple parts of the clitoris, much like the feminist self-help movement did beginning in the 1970s. By labeling the female genitals in detail, feminists sought for women to have more control over and knowledge of their bodies, not just that dictated by the dominant medical profession. However, in doing this the genitals are also made more visible and are able to be placed under scrutiny, as designer vaginas are seen as "fixes" to deformations of the female genitals.

From texts on female anatomy that labeled only certain genital parts and viewed them as a variation of male genitalia to feminists labeling three or more parts of the clitoris, texts construct the value of the female genitals.[15] Feminist self-help texts constructed female genitals that they felt more accurately represented the female body, its sexuality, and its value. Female genitals have not always been constructed by the ideal model that is represented by the medical professional selling the designer vagina.

The history of cosmetic surgery in the United States has also dramatically shaped the value and idealization of the female body. The rise of the beauty industry, what Elizabeth Haiken calls a "consumer beauty culture," greatly influenced the development of cosmetic surgery in the early 1900s. Beginning in the 1930s, plastic surgeons began to recognize that American women were far more likely than wounded soldiers to spend money on plastic surgery. As a result, women, "specifically middle-aged [and] middle-class," became the first official target of the plastic surgery industry. Standards of beauty, or ideal femininity, were upheld by plastic surgeons and the media alike. Haiken says that "Americans created and participated in a new, visual culture, where appearance seemed to rank ever higher in importance."[16]

In the last twenty-five years, the number of plastic surgeons in the United States has increased fourfold. It is not surprising, then, that cosmetic surgery is one of the fastest growing medical specialties.[17] This period in American history can be seen as a time when there has been increased media attention to women's bodies, especially visually. Currently, American women spend Amore than $20 billion annually on cosmetics alone and many billions more on diets, clothes, hair care, and surgery."[18] Haiken has linked this success to "a direct result of the economic gains women made in the post-World War II years" that allowed them in the 1970s and 1980s to "afford to buy the things they wanted, and among the goods they bought were smoother faces, bigger breasts, and thinner thighs."[19] Debra Gimlin reveals that "Board-certified plastic surgeons performed more than 2.2 million procedures in 1999." She goes on to explain that the most frequently received procedure is liposuction, "performed 230,865 times [in 1999] (up 57 percent since 1996 and 264 percent since 1992) at a cost of approximately $2,000 per patient."[20]

The plastic surgery industry most generally sells sameness, as procedures—including the designer vagina—construct a similar aesthetic, that of the Western ideal. Thus, women of various races and ethnicities routinely have surgery to embody this particular Westernized ideal. For instance, Kathryn Pauly Morgan describes how Asian women and girls are having cosmetic surgery to make their eyes rounder and their noses higher, while African-American women are bleaching their skin and Jewish women are having reductions in their noses.[21] Eugenia Kaw argues that Asian-American women who seek eyelid reductions and heightened nose bridges have internalized "racial ideology that associates their natural features with dullness, passivity, and lack of emotion" as they partake in the Western feminine ideal.[22] The idealized femininity of Western culture is imparted upon many women's bodies. Ninety percent of all cosmetic surgery patients are women.[23] Thus, cosmetic surgery is a growing industry and one that has contributed to the development of the designer vagina as more and more areas of the woman's body are becoming areas of cosmetic change.

But for whom is this cosmetic change being done? Heteronormative language and assumptions predominate discourse on designer vaginas. In describing how "tight" to make the woman's vagina in vaginal rejuvenation, one cosmetic surgeon tells a popular woman's magazine, "I give most women's vaginas a two-finger diameter, which is the width of the average penis."[24] The heteronormative language of the designer vagina is reflective of the dominant cultural ideals that encourage women to perform ideal femininity through cosmetic surgery. In the following section we will show the importance of feminist discourses on cosmetic surgery, which explore the role of agency in a woman's choice to undergo surgery to alter her physical body. Because, in seeking cosmetic surgery, there is not only a need to satisfy a male partner but also a need to satisfy an image of oneself.

## FEMINISM AND THE DESIGNER VAGINA

Feminist theorists have commented extensively on cosmetic surgery and what its implications are for the individual woman and for society. Most agree that the upholding of normative and idealized images of femininity and the female body is problematic. Sandra Lee Bartky argues that Michel

Foucault's 1977 text *Discipline and Punish* is crucial to analyzing the state of femininity in modern U.S. society. Bartky believes that the idealized conceptions of femininity construct the barriers of what a female body can become. She states that this Adisciplinary project of femininity is a 'set-up,'" creating a system where "virtually every woman who gives herself to it is destined in some degree to fail."[25] The boundaries of acceptable femininity continually and gradually change, and the project of embodying ideal femininity will never succeed.

This same struggle to define acceptable bodies can be found in the "abject zones" that Judith Butler speaks of in *Bodies that Matter*. These zones are the ideas about our bodies that lead us to think: I would rather die than be fat (or have too small or too large breasts or have long labia). Butler says that the individual "fantasizes [these zones] as threatening its own integrity."[26] As the trends in body projects come and go, the boundaries of the abject zones are always changing, leaving the woman's body potentially always flawed and in need of cosmetic surgery or some other body project. For Bartky, this woman is "the inmate of the Panopticon, a self-policing subject, a self committed to a relentless self-surveillance." Bartky, much like De Beauvior in *The Second Sex*, believes that disciplinary powers are enacted upon women daily in the form of patriarchy.[27]

Quite similarly, Kathryn Pauly Morgan argues what she calls the "Three Paradoxes of Choice," noting that "these choices [to obtain cosmetic surgery] can confer a kind of integrity on a woman's life," yet they "are likely to embroil her in a set of interrelated contradictions."[28] For instance, cosmetic surgery routinely upholds normative societal ideals of bodies, particularly the ideal female body in a white, Western context. Thus, Morgan contends that empowerment language, which is often used to market cosmetic surgery, stands not to empower but to dominate, leaving the recipient of cosmetic surgery at the mercy of the *Other*—the boyfriend, husband, coworker—or, in other words, what she calls "colonized."[29] Morgan contends that the cosmetic surgery recipient is deviant at any point, both for getting cosmetic surgery and for not getting cosmetic surgery. Likewise, Morgan believes that the presence and use of technology is increasing and normalizing in U.S. culture so that a woman is expected to use the technologies available.[30] As a result, Morgan's final paradox states that if the recipient of cosmetic surgery does not use every available means to better herself—to conform to idealized femininity—she is once again deviant.

However, Kathy Davis argues, in contrast to Morgan, that the choice to undergo cosmetic surgery has as much to do with the individual and the connection that the individual sees between her physical self (body) and her mental self (mind). This "embodied subject" is an agent in her own right negotiating this dichotomy. Davis sees the ability to take control of one's body as a potential point of liberation. She states, "Cosmetic surgery can provide the impetus for an individual woman to move from a passive acceptance of herself as nothing but a body to the position of a subject who acts upon the world in and through her body. It is in this sense that cosmetic surgery can, paradoxically, provide an avenue toward becoming an embodied subject rather than an objectified body."[31] For Davis, it is possible that the choice to obtain cosmetic surgery can be about gaining agency, not losing it.

Similar to Davis, Debra Gimlin investigates the cosmetic surgery industry through interviews with both cosmetic surgery recipients and doctors. Gimlin, too, finds the connection of the body and mind central to the woman's discussion of why she made the choice to undergo cosmetic surgery. Gimlin explains that many of the women she interviewed "are using plastic surgery to tell a story about themselves."[32] With such a focus on body projects in Western culture, it is not surprising that Gimlin found that for the women she spoke with, a flawed body often equaled a flawed character.[33] For many women there is a desire, however unsuccessful cosmetic surgery may be in fulfilling it, to obtain surgery in order to improve the self and self-image, to resolve internal problems through bodily means. Gimlin also recognizes larger societal forces at play in the choice to have surgery. She believes that the women obtaining cosmetic surgery are "attempting to make out as best they can within a culture that limits their options."[34]

Within feminist discourse on cosmetic surgery there is the dilemma between representing and respecting the agency of women and recognizing that the scope of their agency is being predetermined by societal forces. Therefore, we assert that the concept of *constrained agency* best negotiates this dilemma. As Gimlin suggests, women who obtain a designer vagina are agents negotiating their experiences within the constructs of a given society. These women seeking surgery experience the contradictions that Morgan has observed as well as the subjectivity that Davis has theorized. This hybrid effect, this constrained agency, is the ultimate outcome.

## DESIGNER VAGINAS IN POPULAR MEDIA

Many magazines and newspapers have addressed the topic of the designer vagina in recent years. They each depict the designer vagina in a way that contributes to the evolving discourse on these cosmetic surgery procedures. For instance, in *Nerve Magazine*, Lisa Carver states that "We [women] could, by harnessing his [Dr. Matlock's] 'laseroscopy' machine, control our vagina."[35] What appears most obvious here is the language of control. The woman with access to cosmetic surgery takes control of her body via technology. The increase in the availability of technology has, therefore, given people the ability to alter their bodies and, as Carver believes, to become empowered to take control of their bodies. Knowledge about designer vaginas is produced, but by whom and for whom? Carver is suggesting that women take the knowledge created by medical technologies and use it to improve their own personal power. In this sense, the laseroscopy machine, as much as the cosmetic surgery, is what gives *control* to the woman. As a result, the woman and the machine are paramount in this representation and the machine is a tool used to provide the woman agency over her body. In Carver's statement, she also makes an endorsement for cosmetic surgery. In effect, she is suggesting that vaginal surgery is an effective way to get *control* over an unruly part of one's body: the vagina. In this way, the vagina is situated as a problematic part of the body needing to be *controlled*.

In an article in *Elle Canada*, author Diane Peters critiques images of the ideal female genitals. She states, "Glance at any porn mag, at least in North America, and the *ideal vagina* is usually perfectly proportioned. The outer labia are plump and smooth, the inner lips are never bigger than the outer, and the clitoral body is small and tidy."[36] This represents the trimming of excess, a reduction of the female body. The ideal female body is represented as slim, and this ideal is represented in vaginal aesthetics, as well. Simone Weil Davis refers to this phenomenon as the "clean slit."[37] The clean slit is the female genitals made to be minimal—the labia are reduced, the vaginal canal is narrowed, and the clitoral hood is reduced or removed. What this means is that the female genitals, like the female body in much popular media, take up less space. By taking up less space, the female genitals are further controlled and made absent in the world. In a historical moment where the embodiment of space often denotes power, we believe that this reduction can also represent a reduction of power for the female body.

Other popular magazines, such as *Playgirl, Harper's Bazaar, New Woman, Woman's Own,* and *Cosmopolitan,* have publicized the designer vagina within their pages. Designer vaginas are said to "work wonders" in Carrie Havranek's article in *Cosmopolitan.*[38] However, some authors aren't as willing to tout the designer vagina without a critical eye. Many of the other magazines contained articles in which doctors, who perform designer vagina surgeries, as well as their satisfied patients were interviewed, but which nonetheless included a short blurb about "not obsessing" over one's genitals and suggested nonsurgical alternatives. For instance, in the *Harper's Bazaar* article entitled "Designer Laser Vaginoplasty," the unnamed author offers some "intimate advice," which informs the reader that she can also do Kegel exercises to tighten the vaginal walls if she does not want surgery.[39] This tells us that despite the buzz around these surgeries, there is still apprehension from at least some authors who investigate designer vaginas.

In contrast to depictions of the "clean slit" is Jennifer Howze's "Vagina 101: What's Normal and What's Not" featured in the October 2005 issue of *Seventeen Magazine*. Unlike the many popular perceptions of the female genitals as deformed in some way, this article, in a magazine geared toward teenaged girls, views the female genitals as less problematic. For instance, one section shows the pictures of two women's genitals—one with shorter labia and the other with labia minora longer than the labia majora—and says, "Length, width and color of the labia minora and labia majora vary from girl to girl. It's also fine if the two sides don't match." The caption of the picture professes that "These are both normal." The article also confronts the issue of vaginal tightness (tightening is a typical designer vagina procedure). The author says that the vaginal walls can be either loose or tight and suggests Kegel exercises that strengthen vaginal muscles, not surgery.[40] Not surprisingly, this issue of *Seventeen* was pulled from the shelves in at least one of the grocery stores in a multistate chain in our area and likely in other areas, as well. This tells us that articles where women are told that their genitals are worthy of fixing are acceptable public information, but when women are shown pictures of their genitals and told that "these are normal," something deviant is seen to have occurred. If the United States is, indeed, a culture of body projects, then the idea that women are told that their bodies are *not* in need of a project is a counterculture move. Although the article in *Seventeen* does not specifically address designer vaginas, the implications are that such designer vagina surgeries, like labia reductions and vaginal tightening, are not necessary and that there are other solutions besides surgery.

Similarly, Debra Olliver on Salon.com provides a critical examination of vaginal surgeries and alteration. Olliver begins by citing the narratives of women who obtained a designer vagina and are pleased with their choice and the results. She follows with an interview with Dr. Matlock, who views his work as a rejection of the focus on women's genitals as purely reproductive organs and insists designer vaginas are a focus on the woman as more, as a sexual being. Although this view of designer vaginas is compelling, Olliver goes on to cite critics who stress the risks involved—"hemorrhage, infection, loss of sensitivity, lingering pain from nerve damage." She also notes that the medical need for designer vaginas is only present in very few women and that the main effect that designer vaginas create is a more youthful aesthetic. Furthermore, Dr. Matlock says that the tightening procedure is often done for male partners, to create a youthful vagina so that men won't stray. What Olliver argues is that although many women are very pleased with their choice to get designer vaginas, they are still partaking in an oppressive system of male dominance.[41]

The designer vagina is constructed in popular media as a blending together of the language of feminism with the focus on the body as representative of the self that can always be improved upon, especially surgically. This is indicative of the Western liberal tradition that focuses on the individual as well as the American ideal of progress and constant improvement. However, the designer vagina is not critiqued in U.S. culture with the same ferocity as other female genital surgeries, such as the cultural practice of female circumcision involving primarily African women. In the final section of this chapter, we show that the rhetoric and overall image in the United States of the empowered woman who seeks the socially acceptable designer vagina procedure are in stark contrast with the popular representations of the African woman who chooses to be circumcised or is circumcised in her culture, even though these procedures themselves are quite comparable.

## A CULTURAL COMPARISON

Comparisons have been drawn between designer vaginas and female circumcision by scholars such as Simone Weil Davis and Leslye Obiora. We argue that designer vaginas are procedures that in many ways mimic those of female circumcision. Both procedures vary (there are as many as five types of female circumcision) and may involve the cutting of the female genitals and the minimizing or elimination of the labia and/or the clitoris. How is the line of differentiation drawn between designer vaginas and female circumcision?

The view in Western discourses of female circumcision as a homogenous, "mutilating" practice suggests a comparison to designer vaginas, which are viewed in a contrasting light. For designer vagina recipients, Davis recognizes this comparison through the desire of patients for sameness, the "clean slit." She says, "the single favored look for these 'designer vaginas' is 'the clean slit.'"[42] As previously discussed, the "clean slit" is the trimmed-back genitalia—smaller, more even pigmentation, and symmetrical structure. Likewise, Davis reports that the doctors she visited "explained to me that the ideal look for labia minora was not only minimal and unextended but also symmetrical, 'homogenously pink,' and 'not wavy.'"[43] Davis draws attention to the photographs of patients displayed on doctors' Web sites and the lack of uniqueness and individuality present in their genitalia.

The "clean slit" is also representative of female circumcision procedures, many of which have the goal of that very aesthetic—from trimming to complete removal of exterior genitalia. Davis cites a group of Egyptian mothers talking about female circumcision and the importance of not having anything "floppy" in the genital area.[44]

The homogenization of African women in U.S. discourse shapes the representations of female circumcision procedures. Leslye Obiora stresses the heterogeneity of not only the procedures of female circumcision but also the cultural milieu in which they are performed. Female circumcision, Obiora states, can be separated into four procedures: pricking the clitoris to shed a few drops of blood; removal of the clitoral hood; excision or clitorectomy; and finally, infibulation, the removal of the outer genitalia.[45] Due to the range of procedures and the various conditions in which they may be performed, the side-effects can vary dramatically, from minor to fatal. In contrast to most U.S. discourses, Obiora states that of the possible sexual side-effects, "Neither sexual frigidity nor the absence of pleasurable sensation at the clitoris can be conclusively related to female circumcision."[46] Kirsten Bell states that "Ahmandu [an author on female circumcision] argues that many women (herself included) who had sexual experiences prior to excision perceive either no difference or increased sexual satisfaction."[47] Davis also notes the range of motivations for women who choose female circumcision to be "beautification, transcendence of shame, and the desire to conform," not unlike U.S. women seeking elective vaginoplasties.[48] In different countries throughout Africa, variations of female circumcision are practiced with a range of motivations. As Obiora and others here contend, female circumcision is not a homogenous procedure.

Davis goes on to quote Soraya Mire, a Somali woman known for making the film *Fire Eyes*, who recognizes the contradiction in the belief that "Western women cut themselves up voluntarily."[49] This popular distinction between the African and Western practice is also made by Diane Peters in *Elle Canada*, who says that female circumcision differs from the designer vagina because it "isn't voluntary."[50] The question of the voluntary status of the female genital operations and the question of choice in particular can surely be disputed on many grounds, most notably with regard to age. In the United States there is the idea that a young person must be a certain age to consent, though this boundary is obviously blurred when one considers the U.S. practice of male circumcision, for instance. Therefore, consent in the United States is also problematic, as parental desires can often trump those of the child or young adult.[51] Both women in the United States and Africa face constraints upon their agency within their respective cultural constructs that shape the process of making a choice.

Another point of differentiation that is important here is the distinction that is made to uphold the Western woman as the emblem of liberal free choice and individualism over the African woman as passive victim of a "primitive" culture. Eric K. Silverman analyzes this stereotype of the African woman when he states that "critics of FC [female circumcision] portray circumcised women as ignorant, hapless, traumatized victims of a brutal patriarchy. This characterization denies many African women the capacity for agency, decision making, and legitimate consciousness."[52] An African woman's agency is hardly recognized, because she is not viewed as a person who possesses subjectivity or is free to act as an agent in her own right. While the designer vagina recipient is represented as a freely choosing consumer, the African woman in U.S. discourse is represented as having no agency.

Such representations divide the West—particularly the United States—from Africa, constructing gendered ideals of women in Africa as passive, acted-upon victims. Obiora states that Western discourses are continually "informed by misconceived notions of African women as nothing but subjugated and devoid of agency. They are objectified 'only as victims and preyers-upon each other'...in negation of their old traditions of power and strength and nurturance found in the female bonding." As a result, Obiora believes that "Myths about their complacency and passive submission perpetuate the stereotype of the quintessential African woman as a beast of burden."[53] As Silverman notes, female circumcision often is performed by other women. He states, "these rites are largely practiced—and advocated—by women."[54] Thus he argues that the dominant Western view is that:

> African and Muslim women are oppressive and insane; Western culture is enabling and free. They are enslaved to an evil, irrational tradition; we transcend tradition through rationality. They subsume individuality within the collectivity; we applaud the person who stands above the crowd. (55)

In a report for Family Health International, Kim Best says, "Many women believe that FGC (female genital cutting) ensures that they will be accepted by their community. They do not know that it is not practiced in most of the world."[56] The impression is that African women are cultural dupes that are not only subjected to their culture but to each other. However, we believe that, like American women seeking designer vaginas, African women are doing their best to get by within a cultural context presenting real constraints.

When U.S. discourses about female circumcision and designer vaginas are put in conversation with each other, the boundaries constructed between them begin to blur. The task in U.S. discourse of separating female circumcision and designer vaginas symbolizes a larger, sustained *othering* of Africa. As J. A. Mbembé states, representations of African culture in U.S. discourses situate Africa as the abject, making the subjectivity of the U.S./West possible. In Western eyes, Africa represents "all that is incomplete, mutilated, and unfinished."[57] This chapter serves not only as a comparison of U.S. discourses of female circumcision and designer vaginas, but as a rejection of the othering of Africa by the West. Thus, the projection of designer vaginas in popular media as a U.S./Western concept of undiminished agency and idealized femininity is made possible in part by the presence of an Other, the image of the circumcised African female who is devoid of agency and sexual subjectivity. This artificial boundary between designer vaginas and female circumcision ignores both the similarities of the procedures and the constrained agency possessed by both groups of women.

## CONCLUSION

Through an examination of the female genital cosmetic surgery procedures called designer vaginas, we have shown how they contribute to the fabrication of the female body in contemporary U.S. culture. Designer vaginas are purported to represent what an "acceptable" female body should look like, reshaping the boundaries of idealized femininity and creating a new aesthetic ideal for the female genitals. This chapter has also attempted to examine the procedures of female circumcision in Africa as they are understood in a U.S. context in comparison to designer vaginas. Furthermore, we have shown that what is ultimately necessary for the presence of one is the presence of the other: The designer vagina is normalized in comparison to female circumcision.

However, what remains consistent throughout this analysis is the importance of constrained agency in framing how individual women experience their designer surgeries. In this essay, we have reformulated the binary model of agency for women seeking cosmetic surgery. As women continue to make choices about their bodies, we believe that more surgical procedures will become available and more bodies will be altered; nevertheless, what will be continually asked is whether these procedures are problematic for women and whether rhetorical work represents consumer agency or absences of agency and choice. However, we must challenge this binary analysis to observe the presence of constrained agency and to examine how agency is obtained and exerted within these absences. As boundaries of the mutability of the woman's flesh and blood body are continually challenged by changes in science and technology, how will women continue to negotiate their agency within these shifting boundaries of legitimacy?

## NOTES

1. Anka Radakovich, "Designer Vaginas," *Playgirl*, December 2000, http://www. drmatlock. com/media.htm. Accessed October 14, 2004.

2. Ibid.

3. Kerry McArthy, "I Paid $5,000 for My Designer Vagina," *New Woman Magazine*, http://www.drmatlock.com/media.htm February 2003.

4. Jen Loy, "Pushing the Perfect Pussy," *Fabula* 4, no. 1 (2000): 26.

5. "'Fringe' Plastic Surgery Procedures More Hype than Reality, ASPS Says Fewer than 800 Vaginal Rejuvenation Procedures in 2005," American Society of Plastic Surgeons, Press Release, http://www.plasticsurgery.org/news_room/ press_releases/fringe-procedures.cfm March 15, 2006.

6. Sarah Klein, "Does This Make My Labia Look Fat? Medicine and Marketing Collide below the Belt," *MetroTimes*, http://www.metrotimes.com/editorial/ story.asp?id=7405 March 9, 2005.

7. McArthy, "I Paid $5,000 for My Designer Vagina."

8. Kathryn Pauly Morgan, "Women and the Knife: Cosmetic Surgery and the Colonization of Women's Bodies," *The Politics of Women's Bodies: Sexuality, Appearance and Behavior*, ed. Rose Weitz (New York: Oxford University Press, 2003), 174.

9. Klein, "Does This Make My Labia Look Fat?"

10. Iris Lopez, "Agency and Constraint: Sterilization and Reproductive Freedom among Puerto Rican Women in New York City," *Situated Lives: Gender and Culture in Everyday Life*, ed. Louise Lamphere, Helena Ragoné, and Patricia Zavella (New York: Routledge, 1997), 157.

11. Ibid., 157–58.

12. Alice Domurat Dreger, *Hermaphrodites and the Medical Invention of Sex* (Cambridge, MA: Harvard University Press, 1998), 4.

13. Judith Butler, *Undoing Gender* (New York: Routledge, 2004), 8.

14. David Matlock, "Mission," Laser Vaginal Rejuvenation Institute of Los Angeles, http://www.drmatlock.com. Accessed on August 26, 2005.

15. Lisa Jean Moore and Adele E. Clarke, "Clitoral Conventions and Transgressions: Graphic Representations in Anatomy Texts, c1900-1991," *Feminist Studies* 21, no. 2 (Summer 1995): 264.

16. Ibid., 23, 38, 11, 91-92.

17. Debra L. Gimlin, *Body Work: Beauty and Self-Image in America* (Berkeley: University of California Press, 2002), 76.

18. Ibid., 9.

19. Elizabeth Haiken, *Venus Envy: A History of Cosmetic Surgery* (Baltimore: Johns Hopkins University Press, 1997), 10.

20. Gimlin, *Body Work*, 75.

21. Morgan, "Women and the Knife," 172.

22. Eugenia Kaw, "Medicalization of Racial Features: Asian American Women and Cosmetic Surgery," *Medical Anthropology Quarterly* 7 (1993): 74-77.

23. Gimlin, *Body Work*, 75.

24. Mandy Appleyard and Natasha Courtney-Smith, "Designer Vaginas: Prettying Up What's Down There," *Woman's Own Magazine*, http://www.drmatlock.com/media.htm. Accessed Octobeer 14, 2004.

25. Sandra Lee Bartky, "Foucault, Femininity, and the Modernization of Patriarchal Power," in *The Politics of Women's Bodies: Sexuality, Appearance and Behavior*, ed. Rose Weitz (New York: Oxford University Press, 2003), 29, 33-34.

26. Judith Butler, *Bodies that Matter: On the Discursive Limits of Sex* (New York: Routledge, 1993), 243.

27. Bartky, "Foucault, Femininity," 41-42.

28. Morgan, "Women and the Knife," 171.

29. For Morgan, the concept of "colonized" refers to the dominant patriarchal culture's viewing of the woman's body as "a 'primitive entity' that is seen only as potential, as a kind of raw material to be exploited in terms of appearance, eroticism, nurturance, and fertility," Morgan, "Women and the Knife," 173.

30. Ibid., 175.

31. Kathy Davis, *Reshaping the Female Body: The Dilemma of Cosmetic Surgery* (New York: Routledge, 1995), 113–14.

32. Gimlin, *Body Work*, 80.

33. Ibid., 104.

34. Ibid., 106.

35. Lisa Carver, "Surrender the Pink," *Nerve Magazine*, http://www. drmatlock. com/media.htm. January 2001. Accessed October 14, 2004.

36. Diane Peters, "Viva La Vulva," *Elle Canada*. Accessed October 14, 2004.

37. Davis, *Reshaping the Female Body*, 4.

38. See also the work of Jean Kilborne on women in the media. Jean Kilbourne, *Can't Buy My Love, How Advertising Changes the Way We Think and Feel* (New York: Simon and Schuster, 1999).

39. "Designer Vaginas," *Harper's Bazaar*, November 1998, 10/14/04.

40. Jennifer Howze, "Vagina 101: What's Normal and What's Not," *Seventeen Magazine*, October 2005, 84-85.

41. Debra Olliver, "Designer Vaginas," Salon.com, http://archive.salon.com/sex/ feature/2000/11/14/vagina/print.html. Accessed October 14, 2004.

42. Simone Weil Davis, "Loose Lips Sink Ships," *Feminist Studies* 28, no. 1 (Spring 2002): 7-37, 9-12.

43. Ibid., 15.

44. Ibid, 24.

45. L. Amede Obiora, "Bridges and Barricades: Rethinking Polemics and Intransigence in the Campaign against Female Circumcision," *Case Western Reserve Law Review* 47, no. 2 (Winter 1997): 275-378, 288-89.

46. Ibid, 308.

47. Kirsten Bell, "Genital Cutting and Western Discourses on Sexuality," *Medical Anthropology Quarterly* 19 (2005): 138.

48. Simone Weil Davis, "Loose Lips Sink Ships," 23.

49. Ibid., 22.

50. Peters, "Viva La Vulva."

51. The topic of voluntariness of FGOs on youth is underdeveloped in this chapter and is an important area to be explored in future research.

52. Eric K. Silverman, "Anthropology and Circumcision," *Annual Review of Anthropology* 33 (2004): 419-45, 431.

53. Obiora, "Bridges and Barricades," 303.

54. Silverman, "Anthropology and Circumcision," 429.

55. Ibid., 431.

56. Kim Best, "Is Female Genital Cutting Ethically Justifiable?" Family Health International. *Network*, 21, no. 2: 2001.

57. Ibid., 1.

# NINE

# (Trans) Gendered Fabrications and the Surgery Debates

## SALLY HINES

IN RECENT YEARS TRANSGENDER HAS emerged as a subject of increasing social and cultural interest. Popular representations of transgender are apparent in television dramas, sitcoms and reality shows, while the "trans confessional" is a talk-show staple. Tabloid journalists and magazine feature writers increasingly search for trans people for "real life" stories, and television documentary and broadsheet journalism has focused upon the experiences of both female and male trans people. Transgender characters have had central roles in recent mainstream films, and on-stage, cross-dressing performers such as Eddie Izzard, Lilly Savage and RuPaul draw large audiences. Much of this focus concerns the physical shifts that accompany gender transformations. This chapter examines how the transgendered body is fabricated through surgical practice.[1]

The first section addresses how surgery is centrally positioned within medical and psychological discourses on transgender, which continue to operate within the hypothesis of the "wrong body." Here surgery is located as a solution to "gender dysphoria" in enabling the emergence of the "true" gendered self. I consider the ways in which medical discourse impacts upon transgender identity formations by addressing the role of surgery within transgender narratives of self-identity and in relation to the construction of transgender social identities. Second, I consider debates around (trans) gendered embodiment within transgender studies, and look at how the "wrong body" metaphor is re-presented, rehearsed, and rejected within transgender narratives at a discursive and an individual level.

Finally, the chapter explores the relationship between surgery and constructions of gendered authenticity and addresses collective debates around surgery within transgender communities

Substantively, the chapter draws on findings from an empirical study of transgender practices of identity to explore how surgical procedures are variously understood and practiced in the "everyday." The research was completed in 2004 at the University of Leeds, United Kingdom. Thirty transgendered men and women were interviewed over a nine-month period in 2002. Thirteen participants were trans men and seventeen were trans women, ranging in age from twenty-six to seventy-one years old.[2] Participants were at different stages of transition, and the sample included people who use hormone therapy and/or a range of surgical modifications as well as those who reject these interventions. All of the participants resided in the UK. While some participants used pseudonyms, others wished to be known by their own names. Theoretically and substantively the chapter positions gender reconstructive surgical practices as a site of contestation. I suggest that understandings and practices of the surgically fabricated body are contingently situated alongside divergent transgendered experiences and identity formations.

## CONSTRUCTING THE "WRONG BODY" IN MEDICAL DISCOURSE AND PRACTICE

Medical and psychological studies have constructed particular ways of thinking about transgender. Moreover, medical and psychological discourses continue to inform social, cultural, and legal understandings of transgender. The theoretical shifts that accompanied the increasing acceptance of reconstructive surgery from the late 1950s onward strengthened the role of the medical practitioner. Benjamin's *Transsexual Phenomenon*[3] and Green and Money's *Transsexualism and Sex Reassignment*[4] introduced the notion of "gender" into discourses of transsexuality, and "gender" came to be recognized independently of "sex." As Ekins and King explain: "If gender is immutable, even though psychologically produced, and if harmony between sex and gender is a precondition of psychic comfort and social acceptability, it 'makes sense' to achieve harmony by altering the body."[5] Thus it was believed that surgery enabled the "true" self to emerge and most practitioners aligned with this narrative. From the early 1970s, the concept of "gender dysphoria" was developed in medical writing. "Gender dysphoria" suggests that those seeking hormone therapy or surgery have been born, and so are living, in the "wrong" body.

By the late 1970s, surgical procedures had become the orthodox method of "treatment" for gender dysphoria.[6] Contemporary medical perspectives continue along a biologically based line; as the 1996 report for the UK Parliamentary Forum on Transsexualism illustrates: "The weight of current scientific evidence suggests a biologically based, multifactoral aetiology for transsexualism."[7] Though later medical insights represent a more complex understanding of transgender practices than were offered within founding medical perspectives, there remain serious problems in the correlation of transgender and biological or psychological pathology. The epistemological power of medical discourse has thus worked to structure specific etiologies of transgender. Significantly, the concept of "gender dysphoria" remains a key classificatory term within medical discourse and practice. From its inception in the 1970s, then, the concept of "gender dysphoria" has guided understandings of, and practices toward, transgender people. Therefore, it is not surprising that the central tenet of the concept—dissonance between sex (the body) and gender identity (the mind)—figures large in many trans narratives. Research participant Bernadette reflected this in reply to my question, "What are the most important changes transition has brought?":

> Before I transitioned, I had become terrified of mirrors. I couldn't look at myself. I was absolutely horrified looking at myself and this was completely resolved. [...] These are the things which have changed, and made me feel what I am. They are the external manifestations that balance. (Bernadette, age seventy-one)

Corresponding with the concept of gender dysphoria, Bernadette positions her pretransition body as the "wrong" vehicle in which her essential self was trapped. Surgical "correction" is subsequently related as the means through which her authentic gender is released. In her discussion of male to female (MtF) autobiography, Stone shows how accounts of the "wrong body" lie at the heart of many personal accounts of transition:

> [T]hey go from being unambiguous men, albeit unhappy men, to unambiguous women. There is no territory between. Further, each constructs a specific narrative moment when their personal sexual identification changes from male to female. This moment is the moment of neocolporraphy—that is, of gender reassignment or "sex change" surgery.[8]

Although the significance placed upon a congruent relationship between gender identity and bodily appearance is reflected by some participants in my research, the desire for surgery is rarely articulated as a straightforward manifestation of gender dysphoria. The only participant to directly relate the "wrong body" experience was Cheryl, age forty-five who, in answer to my question "How do you describe your gender identity?," replied "female trapped in a male body." Significantly, Cheryl had sought medical advice from her doctor only four months before our interview and was still waiting for her first appointment with a psychiatrist. Epstein's application of a Foucauldian analysis is useful for understanding the influence of a medical model upon transsubjectivities. Through medical surveillance the "patient" is viewed as a special type of person, and individual experience is lost as the person emerges as a "medical type."[9] Thus personal accounts are written into medical discourse, which converts "unclear subjectivity into an interpretable text, which takes precedence over the fragments of human experience."[10] Power is transferred from the "speaking subject" to the "expert"[11] to sustain a "regime of truth."[12] In this way, medical case studies do not simply "record," but work to "produce" knowledge and subjective understandings of the self. Much debate within transgender studies has thus been concerned with addressing the contradiction between a constructionist analysis of transgender and the representation of a fixed identity within many transgender autobiographies.

## THEORIZING THE "WRONG BODY" IN TRANSGENDER NARRATIVES

A central question for Prosser in *Second Skins* is how to theorize sex, gender, and identity in the light of continued transsexual demand for reconstructive surgery. He suggests that the "wrong body" narrative reflects a genuine transsexual emotion:

> My contention is that transsexuals continue to deploy the image of wrong embodiment because being trapped in the wrong body is simply what transsexuality feels like. If the goal of transsexual transition is to align the feeling of gendered embodiment with the material body, body image—which we might be tempted to align with the imaginary—clearly already has a material force for transsexuals. The image of being trapped in the wrong body conveys this force. It suggests how body image is radically split off from the material body in the first place, how body image can feel sufficiently substantial as to persuade the transsexual to alter his or her body to conform to it. The image of wrong embodiment describes most effectively the experience of pretransition (dis)embodiment: the feeling of a sexed body dysphoria profoundly and subjectively experienced.[13]

Yet it has been widely acknowledged that, in order to gain access to hormone therapy or surgical procedures, trans people frequently reproduce the officially sanctioned etiology of transsexualism, that of gender dysphoria.[14] Indeed, in the 1970s, Stoller acknowledged this process, remarking: "Those of us faced with the task of diagnosing transsexualism have an additional burden these days, for most patients requesting 'sex change' are in complete command of the literature and know the answers before the questions are asked."[15]

Subsequently, medical professionals have suggested that trans people may "distort their autobiographies (and) tend to be less than honest about their personal histories."[16] As Stone remarks: "This raises several sticky questions, the chief two being: Who is telling the story for whom, and how do the storytellers differentiate between the story they tell and the story they hear?"[17] Thus the "wrong body" narrative may be seen to be medically constructed and internalized as a means to an end: "The idea has been imposed upon transpeople by those who control access to medical technologies and have controlled discourses about transpeople. Some individuals may believe or come to believe that they are in the wrong body or at least use language that imparts the same meaning [...]."[18] In the following quotation from our interview, research participant Gabrielle illustrates how this process may work:

G: If you see a doctor for an hour once every three months and they go "how are you?"and you go "I'm fine." And they go "any issues?" you go "no." "Cos you want what they've got to give you and so you quickly learn the script as people call it, for what you should say and not say. And I think people buy into that, people do say these things that the doctors need to hear to tick off on the form to make you eligible.

S: And what are those things?

G: "I'm a woman trapped in a man's body" or "A man trapped in a woman's body." "I've known always," you know, those sort of things, the things that people say. (Gabrielle, age forty-five)

Gabrielle's narrative connects with Shapiro's argument that "[o]ne cannot take at face value transsexuals' own accounts of a fixed and unchanging (albeit sex-crossed) gender identity, given the immense pressure on them to produce the kinds of life histories that will get them what they want from the medical-psychiatric establishment."[19] The extent to which trans people continue to research diagnostic guidelines is illustrated in the Harry Benjamin "Standards of Care," which formulate the "professional consensus about the psychiatric, psychological, medical, and surgical management of gender identity disorders."[20] The document details the means by which trans people may find "new gender adaptations," stating that "both genders may learn about "transgender phenomena from studying these 'Standards of Care,' relevant lay and professional literatures about legal rights pertaining to work, relationships, and public cross-dressing."[21]

Questions about the impact of a medical model on trans subjectivities brings to mind Foucault's writing on the body. For Foucault, the body is constructed through power: "The body is directly involved in a political field; power relations have an immediate hold upon it; they invest it, mark it, train it, torture it, force it to carry out tasks, to perform ceremonies, to emit signs."[22] Thus subjects are produced through discourses of the body. Complicity with a medical model of transgender both supports and para-doxically challenges Foucault's notion of the "docile body," which is a "direct locus of control" produced by external power. Thus, while the "wrong body" hypothesis can be seen as a discourse that produces its sub-ject, the self-conscious repetition of the "wrong body" narrative can be read as an agency-driven process whereby trans people employ knowledge as power. Foucault's later work is more relevant to this interplay between structure and agency. In discussing "techniques of the self," Foucault cre-ates a space for agency by examining the relationship between external power and subjectivity.[23] From this point, the notion of the "wrong body" can be conceptualized as a rehearsed narrative that is consciously repeated as a means to an end. Yet rehearsed narratives are not only characteristic of transsexual stories, as Shapiro acknowledges:

> To take the problem one step further, the project of autobiographical reconstruction in which transsexuals are engaged, although more focused and motivated from the one that all of us peruse, is not entirely different in kind. We must all repress information that creates problems for cultur-ally canonical narratives of identity and the self, and consistency in gender attribution is very much a part of this.[24]

Within medical understandings of transgender, then, the state of gender dysphoria is relieved through surgical practices. Thus the body and gender identity are synchronized to signpost the analogous gendered "self." Subsequently, medical culture may be seen to have constructed the trans-sexual subject who internalizes the discourse of the "wrong body." However, for many participants in my research the wrong body narrative was deeply unsatisfactory. I asked research participant Rebecca, age fifty-five, how she felt about the wrong body metaphor: "It's [transition] been a progression. It's never been fixed from the outset and I've never had those overwhelming feelings of being in the wrong body. There's always been flu-idity in my feelings." In the following quotation, Amanda presents an explicit critique of the "wrong body" and, like Rebecca, suggests that gender transition is more complex than this metaphor indicates:

The way in which some people talk about being born in the wrong body is such a cliché and to come back to components, we all have a male and a female component. [...] So "wrong body," that's a plumbing job. That's nothing to do with the core person I am, what makes me a person. (Amanda, age forty-five)

For these participants, gender identity formation is a nuanced process, which does not necessarily signify movement across a gender binary. In the following quotation, Del attempts to work through these complexities:

[...] the wrong body stuff does bother me. I think a lot of it is that our culture is wrong, and if our culture was more accepting of gender diversity, would we need to (have surgery)? You know, if men could wear make up and dresses, and for women if there was no glass ceiling, would it be necessary? [...] (Del, FtM age forty-four)

Like Del, Gabrielle raises the question of whether surgery would be necessary in a society that was accepting of gender diversity:

There is something that people have said, it's what I call the "desert island syndrome." If you were on a desert island and there was no one else to see you, would you still have the operation?" And I've said "well, I think I would" but I don't know if I'd never seen a woman's body whether I'd still have felt that, who can say? We can't know what it would be like to be brought up in a bubble. (Gabrielle, MtF, age forty-five)

While the narrative of the "wrong body" is repeated to gain surgical reconstruction, the demand for surgery may be seen to be an outcome of social and cultural investments in a gender binary system. Although some transsexual narratives reflect the desire for a meeting of the gendered body and mind, it is difficult, then, to detach the demand for surgery from medical culture. Although the majority of participants in my research speak of gender transition as a fluid process, which does not necessarily represent a straightforward shift across the gender binary, the gender binary system itself means that people who are gender ambiguous frequently face social and cultural discrimination and hostility. Body modifications may thus bring an increased level of safety and emotional ease as bodily appearance and gender identity meet to confer with normative assumptions. In this way, Del says of his use of hormones, "It made my life easier. It made my passage through the city and the world smoother and less dangerous."

Body modification through the use of hormones and/or surgery, then, can bring security within a culture that is hostile to gender ambiguity. As Nataf states, "Very few people can cross-live, get employment successfully and be safe in the streets without hormones and some surgery."[25] As such, the "wrong body" narrative can be analyzed as a rehearsed narrative that is consciously repeated as a means to an end–that being cultural acceptance. For Stone, though, there is a high price to pay for gender normativity: "The highest purpose of the transsexual is to erase him/her, to fade into the "normal" as soon as possible. . . . What is gained is acceptability in society. What is lost is the ability to authentically represent the complexities and ambiguities of lived experience [. . .]."[26] She proposes that analyses of transgender move away from the wrong body paradigm in order to negotiate "the troubling and productive multiple permeabilities of boundary and subject positions that intertextuality implies."[27] With these points in mind, the following sections of this chapter draw further upon my research data to explore the complexities and ambiguities in the body narratives of participants. Subsequent sections address the role surgery plays in reconciling self and social identity, and explore debates about surgery and the construction of gendered authenticity within transgender communities.

## SELF-IDENTITY, SOCIAL IDENTITY, AND SURGICAL PRACTICES

While Prosser's emphasis upon wrong embodiment reinforces Descartes' mind/body split, Merleau-Ponty's work offers an alternative framework through which to explore issues of transgender embodiment.[28] In challenging the duality of mind/body, Merleau-Ponty theorizes the intersections between the material body and the phenomenological realm to explore how the body is consciously experienced. The "corporeal schema" indicates how the embodied agent is positioned between the subjective and the social world. For Merleau- Ponty, embodiment is not necessarily a conscious state, but may be experienced as an "inner sense," which influences our bodily actions and responses.

The intersections of the subjective, material, and social were apparent in this research when participants discussed surgery as a way of reconciling self-identity and social identity. Dan, for example, spoke of the fissure between his gender identity and self-bodily image prior to transition:

> I just spent my whole life in front of the mirror thinking "where's my stubble?" and it was always good for me that my figure was very up and down and I was small on top. But I was always very concerned that I looked as boyish as possible. That's what was important to me. And when I looked in the mirror it was always, "how masculine do I look?" (Dan, FtM, age thirty-seven)

For Dave (age twenty-six), masculinity was also strengthened through chest surgery: "Surgery was very important [. . .]. I had to bind myself up everyday and, apart from the discomfort, I just felt they shouldn't be there [...]. For Phillip, age forty-two, taking hormones has reinforced his masculine identity: "Well, I've felt a lot more solid. I've put on a stone in weight. Yeah, I feel more male physically."

In articulating the complex relationship between embodiment and gender identification, these narratives resonate with Freud's notion of "bodily ego,"[29] whereby our sense of "self" develops through our sense of the body. Grosz conceptualizes this as a "psychical map," through which our formation of "self" involves a psychical image of our body.[30] While the understandings and experiences of surgery of several participants in this research suggest that the material body "matters," as Nataf argues: "The achieved anatomy is a way of relieving the confusion and anxiety, and the body is a point of reference, not a nature."[31] In thinking about surgical reconstruction as a "cosmetic" procedure, Halberstam offers a useful way of disengaging the desire for surgery from medical discourses of the wrong body:

> The reason that I say it's cosmetic surgery is because people are always changing their bodies, especially in America. I suppose that if we considered what we're now calling transsexual surgery as cosmetic, maybe we would take the stigma away. Maybe we wouldn't see it as the complete, pathological rearrangement of identity, even if it's experienced as such. Maybe we'd begin to see it is a way of organizing your body to suit your image of yourself. And then we wouldn't have to have this whole therapeutic intervention, where people are saying, "Why do you want to become a man? What's wrong with you?" You could say, "Because I prefer the way a penis looks on my body to the way a vagina looks on my body."[32]

Although chest surgery is a relatively simple and available procedure, the reconstruction of a penis through phalloplasty surgery is a complex and expensive practice. Significantly, only one of the male participants in this research had had phalloplasty. For most of the men interviewed, phalloplasty was seen as a risky and unsatisfactory procedure. Greg, for example, says:

> Phalloplasty is still far from perfect, and at the moment I don't want it. Not because I don't want to have a penis, but I feel it's still not a penis, it doesn't do anything. I mean some do look quite good but there's no surgeon yet who will create a fully functioning sensual, so you can have sexual pleasure, penis through which you can pee and which is erectile. It's just not possible so I just feel it's a massive risk to take 'cos it's a massive procedure. (Greg, FtM, age forty-four)

Other men, such as Dan, question the relationship between masculine identity and male body parts: "I cannot see that having a phalloplasty will then make me say, 'right that's it, I'm a man.' [...] I am a man. I'm the man that I want to be."

So far this chapter has explored the ways in which medical, social, and cultural investments in a gender binary system impact upon the demand for gender reassignment surgical practices. Research data has shown that while some participants view surgery as an important means of reconciling self and social identity, others question and reject the emphasis placed upon a congruent relationship between the gendered body and gender identity within medical and cultural discourse. Yet, as the final section now moves on to address, pressures faced by trans people to change their bodies through surgery may also come from within transgender communities.

## SURGERY DEBATES WITHIN TRANSGENDER COMMUNITIES

While many participants in my research have undergone some surgical procedures in order to bring together bodily appearance and gender identity, others reject surgery. Like Dan, Amanda questions the assumption that surgical reconstruction authenticates gender identity:

> This thing about being complete when you have the op...I don't go with that. I think I'm as complete now as I ever will be. I don't really have any other changes that need to be done that the world needs to know about. My social changes—the side that the world will see—that has now been established and I am supremely comfortable with that. (Amanda, MtF, age forty-five)

Far from being uniformly accepted, then, surgery was viewed as problematic by a significant number of participants. In the following quotation, Rebecca suggests that there is insufficient discussion within transgender communities about the complexities surgical reconstruction may bring:

> One has to worry that there may be people who have gone down the transsexual route and were reassigned, and are having difficulties with that reassignment, who may well have benefitted from a more liberal view. I mean, I have come across one or two transsexuals who are desperately unhappy in their new gender role and it's too late. And that's really sad. And the other problem is that so much of our futures are in the hands of medical professionals and I suspect that many lay people take as read that doctors know best and so therefore "transsexual" is in many ways a medical term; "that's what the doctor says I am." And I wouldn't want to say that people follow it like sheep, but there is a degree of thoughtlessness about possibilities and they fall into that rut, and they don't question it or ask themselves "is this what I really want?" It's just a

solution to what they see as a problem and it's the only one they're offered, so take it or leave it, it's Hobson's choice. (Rebecca, bigendered, age fifty-five)

Like Rebecca, Del suggests that certain issues around surgery are left unspoken within transgender communities:

I think that surgeries are about empowering the doctors, not the patient. I think that very few people are ever really happy. I don't know of any phalloplasty that is problem free, although I'm not saying there aren't, there could well be, but from what I've seen. . . . There's just this continuation and I've seen it happen: "Well, once I get this operation I'll be a real male" [. . .] But I also need to respect the reasons why [...] I'm trying to keep an open mind about it, but I see that right now there's a real trend towards phalloplasty, where it's always been kind of against in FtM groups. It's like now, "That's the icing on the cake" [. . .] But to not problematize these areas, and to not examine them is dangerous is what I believe, and support groups provide a venue for learning a script that is not necessarily true to each person.

Rather than being straightforwardly experienced, then, surgery is a contentious issue within transgender communities. A particular matter of concern raised by research participants is the role of surgery in constructions of gendered authenticity. Subsequently, some participants spoke of a hierarchy whereby surgically reconstructed trans people renounce the self-identified gender of those who do not go down the surgical route. In this way, Rebecca says:

I've had rejection in the past in that sense because I'm not playing the surgery game. I've had transsexuals telling me that I'm not right; "you're not allowed to be like that, you've got to be like us." I can understand where they're coming from, as a transsexual wants to move exclusively from one end of the binary spectrum to the other, and so therefore they have to believe in the binary nature of gender and sex. And so anyone who says "I don't believe in this" is a threat to them. I understand that, but I just found it very disappointing that people who have found their lives very difficult because of feelings of gender dysphoria can't understand where I'm coming from. I can understand Fred Bloggs down the road not understanding where I'm coming from, but for someone who's in a very similar position to myself being prejudiced against me, I do find that quite shocking. I'm sure there is a narrative which goes on in these groups and people learn to play along with rules of that narrative. I suppose the experience that I did have with that group goes to support that in that there was a party line, a three line whip. That to me seems likely to be about protection and safety. If we know who we are and we're all the same, it's safety in numbers. If you've got someone who's a bit different, where does that place us?[33]

Gabrielle also draws attention to a hierarchical politics of identity based upon surgical procedures within some transgender communities: "There's a horrible pecking order amongst trans people, stereotypes, you know, a pyramid of validity against heterosexual cross-dressers with their suitcase in the garage and the box in the loft, and all those horrible ideas, a sort of elite."

These debates illustrate how definitions of gendered authenticity, which are largely constructed in the light of societal discriminatory discourses and practices, may lend themselves to essentialist identity claims that refute the nonnormative identities of others. Support groups run by and for transgender people are identified as a particular arena in which such contentions may arise. Thus Del says:

> You go to a support group and you find exactly how to repeat the narrative which was and may still be a necessary step to get the hormones or to get the surgeries. I think it's social pressure, peer pressure. I think it's the dominant narrative within transsexual communities [...] I feel kinship with transsexual communities because I have a lot of transsexual friends, but in some ways there's a political division between how I think and how they think. I'm critical of a hierarchy in transgendered circles based on what surgery you should have. And I think that sometimes transsexual communities promote those concepts. I found myself being very skeptical. I'm not across-the-board anti-surgery, but I think that if gender wasn't so polarized, if there wasn't such a cultural imperative to be either male or female, that surgery would be less necessary.

Rather than a politics of identity that is based upon notions of gendered authenticity as fabricated through surgery, Del presents a more fluid model of identity, which does not necessarily demand a relation between gender identity and the body:

> I don't think it's [gender identity] linear. I think it's more like if you have [Del draws diagram]. Here we have our source and that's whoever we are and it shoots out in a more kind of radial way, so it's more like a kind of color chart and you can pick all the different colors. [...] So I don't see it as like here you have drag kings and the next step is going to be hormones and the next step is going to be surgery, although sometimes people do that.

Like Del, Rebecca is doubtful of the benefits of genital surgical reconstruction. For Rebecca, rejecting the surgical route of transition has enabled increased gender fluidity. She says:

I suppose my story has changed and matured as time has gone by, and my view of my gender has appeared differently to me at different times. In terms of my place in society now in many ways I feel that I have the best of both worlds. I have an inner peace because I'm more congruent in terms of my external description and internal beliefs, and I can move in society comfortably in that female role on the whole. It has been a struggle and there have been problems along the way, but also by not losing the male side of my being I can call on that [...] I see that as a benefit because I don't live in fear of being acknowledged as a male, or having male characteristics, should I say.

These discussions suggest that while identity is experienced through the body, the relationship between gender identity and the physical body shifts and evolves through transition. Thus my research findings support Nataf's comment that "the form gender identity and role finally take can be more or less fixed or fluid, depending upon the individual."[34]

## CONCLUSION

The notion of the wrong body remains central to medical understandings of, and practices toward, transgender. Within medical culture, surgery is a remedy for gender dysphoria; thus the gendered body and mind are aligned to construct the normative gendered subject. While medical culture understands gender as distinct from biological sex, and, as such, allows for movement across the binary of male/female, the spectrums in-between male and female, such as transgendered, intersexed, bigendered, and androgynous, remain outside of current medical analytical frameworks. Although some theorists within transgender studies propose that the wrong body metaphor is an apt description of transsexual embodiment,[35] others argue that it is a medical construction, and moreover, that the prevalence of the wrong body narrative erases the complexities of transgender experiences and identities.[36]

The body is experienced, managed, and modified through subjective and social understandings of gender. Participants' narratives suggest that surgical procedures are undertaken to reconcile self-identity and social identity, and to ease the difficulties of living within a gender binary system that discriminates against gender ambiguity. Moreover, the demand for surgery is difficult to disentangle from the social and cultural pressures to inhabit a gender-normative body. While many participants altered their bodies through surgical procedures, few narratives of surgery are complicit with the discourse of the wrong body. Rather, the wrong body metaphor is explicitly critiqued by many participants, who speak of gender transition as a more nuanced and complex process. Rather than seeing gender reassignment surgery as an end-point, many participants discuss how their understandings and experiences of embodiment shifted through transition. For some participants, it was unnecessary to align the body and gender identity through surgical reconstruction, yet many spoke of the cultural pressures from both inside and outside transgender communities to do so. These discussions indicate that surgery is a contested issue within transgender communities, particularly in relation to constructions of gendered authenticity.

While the corporeal body is central to transgender sensibilities, this chapter has addressed how transgender identities are constructed and negotiated through and in opposition to medical discourse and practice. The narratives of participants in this research thus suggest that although identity is embodied, experiences of (trans) gender embodiment are fluidly situated and practiced.

## NOTES

1. In this chapter the terms "trans" and "transgender" apply to individuals who have undergone hormone treatment or surgery to reconstruct their bodies, and to those who cross gender in ways that are less permanent. When referring specifically to people who have gone through the medical system for gender reassignment surgery, I use the term "transsexual."

2. "Trans" is an umbrella term that covers all transgender people. In this essay, "trans" is used to refer to transsexual and transgender people.

3. Harry Benjamin, *The Transsexual Phenomenon* (New York: Julian Press, 1966).

4. *Transsexualism and Sex Reassignment*, eds. Richard Green and John Money (Baltimore: Johns Hopkins University Press, 1969).

5. Richard Ekins and Dave King, *Blending Genders: Social Aspects of Cross-Dressing and Sex-Changing* (London: Routledge, 1996), 94.

6. Jason Cromwell, *Transmen and FtMs: Identities, Bodies, Genders and Sexualities* (Urbana: University of Illinois Press, 1999).

7. *Transsexualism: The Current Medical Viewpoint* (1996), www.pfc.org.uk. Accessed September 2003.

8. Sandy Stone, "The Empire Strikes Back: A Posttransexual Manifesto," in *Body Guards: The Cultural Politics of Gender Ambiguity*, eds. Julie Epstein and Kristina Straub ( New York: Routledge, 1991), 286.

9. Julie Epstein, *Altered Conditions: Disease, Medicine and Storytelling* (London: Routledge, 1995), 26.

10. Ibid., 29.

11. Andrew Sharpe, *Transgender Jurisprudence: Dysphoric Bodies of Law* (London: Cavendish Publishing Limited, 2002), 25.

12. Michel Foucault, *Power/Knowledge: Selected Interviews and Other Writings, 1972–1977* (New York: Pantheon, 1980).

13. Jay Prosser, *Second Skins: The Body Narratives of Transsexuality* (New York: Columbia University Press, 1998), 69.

14. See, for example, Richard Green, "Definition and Synopsis of Aetiology of Adult Gender Identity," www.gires.org.uk/Text_Assets/Etiology_Definition, 1969; Stone, "The Empire Strikes Back"; Bernice Hausman, *Changing Sex: Transsexualism, Technology, and the Idea of Gender* (Durham and London: Duke University Press, 1995); Anne Bolin, *In Search of Eve: Transsexual Rites of Passage* (South Hadley: Bergin and Garvey, 1998); and Cromwell, *Transmen and FtMs*.

15. Robert Stoller, "The Transsexual Experiment," *Sex and Gender*, Vol. 11 (London: Hogarth Press, 1975), 248.

16. Leslie Lothstein quoted in Cromwell, *Transmen and FtMs*, 124.

17. Stone, "The Empire Strikes Back," 248.

18. Cromwell, *Transmen and FtMs*, 104.

19. Judith Shapiro, quoted in Zachary Nataf, *Lesbians Talk Transgender* (London: Scarlet Press, 1996), 19.

20. *The Harry Benjamin International Gender Dysphoria Association's Standards of Care for Gender Identity Disorders*, Version Six, 2001.

21. Ibid.

22. Foucault, *The History of Sexuality*, Vol. 1: An Introduction (New York: Random House, 1978), 25.

23. Foucault, *The Use of Pleasure: The History of Sexuality*, Vol. II, trans R. Hurley (New York: Pantheon, 1985).

24. Shapiro quoted in Nataf, *Lesbians Talk Transgender*, 19.

25. Nataf, *Lesbians Talk Transgender*, 43.

26. Stone, "The Empire Strikes Back," 295.

27. Ibid., 297.

28. Maurice Merleau-Ponty, *The Phenomenology of Perception* (London: RKP, 1962).

29. Sigmund Freud, "The Ego and the Id," trans. Strachey et al., *The Standard Edition of the Complete Psychological Works of Sigmund Freud (1953–1965)* (London: Hogarth Press, 1923).

30. Elizabeth Grosz, *Volatile Bodies: Towards a Corporal Feminism* (Bloomington: Indiana University Press, 1994).

31. Nataf, *Lesbians Talk Transgender*, 45.

32. Judith Halberstam, quoted in Nataf, *Lesbians Talk Transgender*, 56.

33. "Fred Bloggs" is the British equivalent of the American "Joe Schmoe."

34. Nataf, *Lesbians Talk Transgender*, 20.

35. Prosser, *Second Skins*.

36. Stone, "The Empire Strikes Back."

TEN

# On Slanderous Words and Bodies-Out-of-Control:

## Hospital Humor and the Medical Carnivalesque

LISA GABBERT AND ANTONIO SALUD II

> Laughter is the best medicine.
> —Traditional proverb

PERHAPS BETTER THAN ANYBODY, PHYSICIANS and other health-care workers understand the vast difference between the ideology of biomedicine and reality. Michel Foucault's *The Birth of the Clinic* initially outlined the biomedical perspective and, since that time, how bodies are controlled, disciplined, monitored, contained, and presented in biomedical contexts has been the subject of vast amounts of research across both the humanities and the social sciences.[1] Most of that research has illustrated how Western biomedical models attempt to achieve complete knowledge/control of the body by routinely objectifying and dehumanizing patients through any number of techniques common to most totalizing institutions, including the regulation of sleep, food, activity, environmental setting, and dress.[2] Although such procedures are done under the guise of disease management—attempting to achieve balance between perceived states of normalcy and dysfunction—past research has revealed that biomedical models constitute a powerful means by which knowledges and ideologies, particularly about gender, race, and other measures of "normal" bodies, are produced and circulated.[3]

But actual human bodies don't always follow institutional scripts and so in practice challenge the Foucauldian ideal of rationalized order. Bodies have ideas of their own—patients don't always follow their doctors' orders, or they do so in novel ways. They also don't necessarily heal in spite of good medical care; they decay or simply die. And as a location for the enactment of life and death, the hospital is stressful, chaotic, and inefficient, despite the posture of rationalization. Moreover, in the ideal biomedical model, doctors are supposed to be competent, caring, omniscient, and omnipotent managers in the production of health. Yet they make mistakes, guess, or are simply incompetent, subverting the ideological model in real life. The discourses produced by totalizing institutions such as hospitals not only affect clients, patients, and inmates but also those who work there. While patients eventually leave the hospital one way or another, medical professionals spend their entire working lives within its walls.[4]

Humor, which is found in a number of high-stress or dangerous occupations, is unsurprisingly an important communicative strategy for doctors and health-care professionals in hospital settings, and we postulate that humor is a primary way of subverting biomedical discourses. Humor occurs particularly in the backstage realms of hospitals such as call rooms, hallways, medical rounds, and curb-side consults. Scholars across a variety of disciplines have previously recognized the prevalence of medical humor.[5] As will be illustrated, medical humor is notoriously off-color, scatological, sexual, or gallows-oriented. Much of this humor is directed at patients, their diseases, their bodies, necessary medical procedures, and even medical workers themselves. To the casual observer, medical humor can appear inappropriate, disrespectful, disciplining, or even cold-hearted. Because of its somewhat disreputable nature, most interpretations in the past have uniformly suggested that medical humor functions to relieve stress, to express hostility toward patients and co-workers, to express irritation at having to provide useless care, or to address the social taboos that physicians routinely break during the course of medical procedures. Importantly, humor and humorous narratives also play an important role in the socialization of medical students.[6]

Folklorist Peter Narváez notes that in spite of—or perhaps because of—its ability to shock, paradoxical juxtapositions of humor and death are on the rise in the modern world, manifested in joke cycles such as Dead Baby jokes, disaster event jokes like those about 9/11, and festive juxtapositions of death in calendar customs and popular culture.[7] Building on this growing awareness of the importance of death, humor, and the body, we utilize Mikhail Bakhtin's notion of carnival laughter to suggest that humor in medical contexts indexes what we call the "medical carnivalesque."[8] Found most obviously in laughter, jokes, and humorous slang but also in asides, insults, and ritual abuse, the medical carnivalesque acknowledges the body as a site of struggle over the production of meaning, mediating the emergent tensions among powerful institutional discourses, profound cultural ideologies, and actual social realities. For Bakhtin, carnival laughter is inherently ambivalent. Drawing on combinations of exaggerated imagery of flatulence and excrement, fertility and sex, gluttony and violence, it mocks, degrades, and destroys but at the same time it is also a source of endless renewal. Given the constant tension between life and death that pervades the hospital environment as well as the totalizing nature of the institution itself, it is not surprising to find a modern form of carnivalesque laughter in this context. Drawing on a variety of resources including literature, published scholarship, collectanea, television, and personal observations, we suggest that the medical carnivalesque indexes an essential but heretofore unrecognized perspective in medical culture, a perspective that tacitly acknowledges the absurdity of the project of modernity, while at the same time participating in it.

## BIOMEDICAL MODELS AND IDEOLOGIES OF CONTROL

The reductionism and impulse toward complete bodily control inherent in contemporary biomedical models evolved from a mingling of Christian traditions and early modern scientific perspectives. Drawing on Rasmussen, George L. Engel notes that early Christianity separated the mind from the body by proscribing the "view of the body as a weak and imperfect vessel for the transfer of the soul from this world to the next."[9] In believing the body as such, what belonged to the body was science and to the mind/soul was religion or spirituality. Coupled with dualism and reductionism in foundational thinkers such as Galileo, Newton, and Descartes, Christianity, Western science, and philosophy profoundly affected the development of modern medicine as a system for the investigation of disease, rather than illness, experience, or suffering.[10]

Today, modern Western biomedicine is what Giddens calls an "expert system."[11] Expert systems, in which people depend on the technological expertise of strangers, are characteristic of late modernity. Indeed, biomedicine is often considered to be modernity's apex. The biomedical system depends heavily on specialized and expert knowledge of disease, meticulous and disciplined scientific reasoning, and the discovery and application of technology in an effort to understand, influence, and manage it. Disease is defined as deviancy from an idealized model of health and is explained by focusing on physiological processes and biochemical mechanisms. "In the narrow biological terms of the biomedical model, this means that disease is reconfigured *only* as an alteration in biological structure or functioning."[12] Origins are sought through a focus on a single, somatic/physical cause. According to this reductionist model, illness is reshaped into disease, symptoms translated into signs, subjective experience expressed as objective data.

The biomedical reductionist model serves as the educational, training, and practicing backbone for physicians, who are an important, embodied contact point with the expert system. Medicine's power relies on its ability to take control of the body by reducing it to parts composed of physiological processes and biological/organic functioning. The medical community does this partly by creating a language that allows it to better understand details and data so that it can find patterns to aid in the diagnosis and eventual treatment of the patient. Part of a physician's responsibility is to transform an ill person into a patient with a disease— that is, into an entity that is objective and scientific in order to lead to a diagnosis and therapy. In other words, "[M]edicine [is characterized] as an ideological system that 'calls' the patient to be an identity that medicine maintains for him; the diagnosis is the most prevalent form of this identity. The ideological work of medicine is to get the patient to accept this diagnostic identity as appropriate and moral."[13] Patient bodies are entextualized, for example, through charts and the case history; here, illness is reduced to particular signs. In the chart and case history, physicians retell patient narratives in a form that identifies patterns and trends by focusing on individual parts, transforming the experience of illness into an authoritative medical history.[14] These numbers become more reliable than the patient him/herself.[15]

The greatest strength of the biomedical model is also its greatest weakness. While a physician can transform a person with an illness into a patient with a disease, s/he may be unable to transform the patient back. The medical model enables the physician to study the body but not necessarily care for the person. The biomedical reductionist model has trained generations of physicians to contemplate and confront disease, but has it trained generations of physicians to address issues of suffering? Eric Cassell writes that nonmedical providers were "shocked to discover the problem of suffering was not directly addressed in medical education. . . . The relief of suffering, it would appear, is considered one of the primary ends of medicine by patients and laypersons, but not by the medical profession."[16] The medical carnivalesque, which often entails laughing at a patient's expense, is one way in which physical suffering is acknowledged by medical consciousness, and from a Bakhtinian perspective it also is one way in which it is conquered.

## THE MEDICAL CARNIVALESQUE

"You gave her what?" asked Fats.

"Thorazine."

Fats burst into laughter. Big juicy laughs rolled down from his eyes to his cheeks to his chins to his bellies, and he said, "Thorazine! That's why she's acting like a chimp. Her blood pressure can't be more than sixty. Get a cuff. Potts, you're terrific. First day of internship, and you try to kill a gomer with Thorazine."[17]

This passage, taken from Samuel Shem's novel *The House of God*, exemplifies the medical carnivalesque. The book satirically tells the story of the inculcation of medical trainees. Here, the intern Potts has mistakenly given an elderly patient improper medication. His supervisor, a seasoned resident commonly known as the Fat Man or Fats, responds with "big, juicy laughter," showers both praise and abuse on Potts by calling him "terrific" while at the same time identifying the patient as a "chimp" and a "gomer." Fats' laughter, the name-calling and abuse, the absurdity of the mistake, and the bulk of Fats' own corporeal being, particularly his "bellies," all suggest the presence of carnivalesque laughter.

Bakhtin's notion of carnivalesque laughter depends on grotesque realism and images of the grotesque body for its effect. The grotesque body is out of control; it is a body that resists closure and exists in the act of becoming.[18] Exaggerated, overabundant, and excessive physical images predominate, including gigantic sexual organs, huge bellies, large noses and other protuberances, the gluttonous consumption of both food and drink, references to ingesting urine and excrement, and images of beatings, bodily dismemberment, blood, disease, and death. By thrusting all that society exalts or idealizes downward into the body's "lower stratum,"[19] carnivalesque laughter mocks and overturns established social orders and offers a mechanism for change, renewal, and rebirth. At the same time, because it renews as it destroys, carnivalesque laugher is inherently ambivalent.

Bakhtin's ideas are entirely applicable to medical contexts, which by definition deal with issues of life and death, control and chaos. Etymologically, the word "carnival" is derived from the word *carne*, which refers to flesh, while the original meaning of "humor" stems from premodern physiology and refers to the four main fluids of the body that determined a person's mood and disposition.[20] As noted above, Western biomedicine not only seeks to know intricate and complex physiological and pathophysiological relationships, but also tries to control them with surgical interventions, medical therapies, and pharmacological interventions. As the patient becomes more ill, physicians attempt to exert more control over basic bodily functions such as breathing, eating, urinating, and defecating. Thus, the grotesque, out-of-control body constitutes a powerful image that counters the modern project of staving off death at all costs. This image calls attention to absolute control as absurd, making mockery of the sacrosanct nature of modern medicine. As a metacommunicative strategy, the use of humor and carnivalesque laughter go directly against the instrumental use of language among medical staff, commenting on and reframing ongoing situations in alternative ways. This is language that is doubly voiced, speaking to official ideologies of medical control while at the same time subverting them for its own purposes.

Degradation is key to grotesque realism, and excrement is the most suitable material for that purpose.[21] Indeed, references to excrement and the anus are so prevalent in medical humor and medical slang that an entire article has been published on the matter.[22] "Bobbing for apples" or "scooping poop," for example, are terms used for the task of removing impacted feces, while a "Code Brown" refers to a patient's fecal incontinence; alternatively it can also mean that a patient needs an enema.[23] As a constant source of work for doctors and as suffering people who are supposed to be treated with utmost respect, patients often are a prime object of degradation. Indeed, the fact that they often are degraded, which is accomplished in the following jokes by relating them to feces or the rectum, suggests their importance in the medical world:

> Q: Doctor, why do you have that thermometer behind your ear?
>
> A: Damn. Some asshole must have my pen.[24]

Doctors might also diagnose patients as having "rectal-cranial inversion"—in other words, the patient has his head up his ass.[25]

The medical carnivalesque mocks and degrades patients, but all participants—including physicians—are potential subjects since flattening hierarchies is an important aspect of humor. A "High Sphincter Tone," for example, is an uptight attending physician, while a "stool magnet" is a doctor who has bad luck when on call.[26] In the example below, doctors, not patients, are the joke's butt:

> Q: What's the difference between a nurse and a toilet seat?
>
> A: A toilet seat only has to deal with one asshole at a time.[27]

References to excrement, however, have multiple functions of which degradation is but one. Eating excrement, for example, conflates what normally are construed to be oppositional bodily processes into ambivalent images that link nourishment, fertility, and life with dismemberment and death.

*Scrubs*, a popular television comedy about physicians-in-training, provides many linkages between ingestion and defecation. In one episode of *Scrubs*, eating and feces are linked by the sardonic comment, "my favorite chips cause anal leakage." In another episode, Carla, a nurse, is ridiculed for carrying around a beaker of urine as she attempts to find its owner. She takes the beaker to the cafeteria and is accused of trying to steal some "apple juice" while a co-worker next in line actually does try to steal apple juice by placing it in several urine beakers. This may not be so far from reality as, indeed, both authors have observed health-care workers using beakers as drinking cups. Robinson also acknowledges the linkage of food and viscera in the following one-liner: "Liver again! Pathology must have had an oversupply this week!"[28] In these examples, ingestion, reproduction, and death are drawn into the same framework, suggesting that these processes are but two sides of the same coin.

The use of billingsgate—that is, foul or profane language, particularly as found in oaths, curses, and *blaison populaire*—also draws heavily on scatological references but for purposes of blasphemy. In the work of Rabelais, the most profane swearing is accomplished by rending apart the body of Christ.[29] In contemporary medical contexts, both patient and physician bodies are torn asunder. In one *Scrubs* episode, the aptly named Dr. Cox, a supervising attending, tells Dr. Kelso, the chief of medicine, "I know that the very idea of you doing a favor for me makes those ass cheeks clinch up so tight that you could shove a lump of coal up there and probably crap out a diamond, right?" In the same episode, Dr. Cox complains that Dr. Kelso was "so far up my ass I can taste Brillo cream in the back of my throat." Rending apart the body of Christ was useful for Rabelais, because Christ was the most sacred body available; as such, its rendering was a most blasphemous act. Both physician and patient bodies are torn verbally apart in medical work contexts, which suggests a kind of sacred nature as to how they are constituted in modern work. Their rending apart contributes to the overall blasphemous thrust of the medical carnivalesque.

Degradation and blasphemous acts create chaos that belies medicine's ability ultimately to take control of the body. And, when bodies cannot be neatly managed, the medical carnivalesque invents absurd procedures to exert control, usually based in the lower body. The bowel prep is one such measure:

> "What is it with this GI workup?" I asked. "She says she's depressed and has a headache."
>
> "It's the specialty of the House," said Fats, "the bowel run. TTB—Therapeutic Trial of Barium."
>
> "There's nothing therapeutic about barium. It's inert."

"Of course it is. But the bowel run is the great equalizer."

"She's depressed. There's nothing wrong with her bowels."

"Of course there's not. There's nothing wrong with her, either."[30]

Another invented procedure is the "required" rectal exam as outlined by Odean: "There are only two reasons *not* to do a rectal exam: 1) the patient has no rectum; 2) the intern has no finger."[31] This constitutes a particularly carnivalesque example, conflating both patient and intern dismemberment with absurdity and lower stratum references. In both cases, the humor underlying the invented absurdity is doubly voiced, speaking to both the kind of control from which modern medicine derives its power while at the same acknowledging that power as fragile and incomplete.

Bodily dismemberment also figures in jokes, many of which target physicians. Although disrespectful, these jokes are not necessarily blasphemous, but they do debase their revered status. One joke based on stereotypes of medical specialties refers to body parts that certain kinds of doctors are perceived not to use or need with any regularity or significance; these are the parts used to "save" an elevator door. The joke complex is told in its entirely; the final exchange concerns hospital administrators, who are often perceived by medical staff as cold-hearted and distant. The fact that the hospital administrator is *not* dismembered is particularly telling in terms of how he/she is perceived in the workplace.

Q: How does a surgeon save the elevator door?

A: Uses his foot.

Q: How does an internist save the elevator door?

A: Uses his hand.

Q: How does an orthopedist save the elevator door?

A: Uses his head.

Q: How does a medical administrator save the elevator door?

A: Uses somebody else.

The medical carnivalesque is also a constant source of renewal and rebirth; hence, references to fertility, birth, exaggerated sexual organs, and other images of sexuality are an essential dimension. In medicine, dialogue and behaviors involving sexuality are plentiful. In Great Britain, for example, a TUBE stands for a Totally Unnecessary Breast Examination.[32] In *The House of God* Dr. Basch and Runt, a sex-obsessed medical intern, have sex with multiple nurses in the same call room simultaneously.[33] Nurses are an unending source of sexual innuendo. There is, for example, the proverbial "theory of action-potential." This is based on a real scientific theory called the action-potential theory, which postulates that the more energy invested in an object, the more potential it has for movement. When applied to nurses, the theory of action-potential is summed up by the proverbial saying "where there's more action, there's more potential," suggesting that in times of much activity, such as the O.R., there is more potential for sex. Robinson also suggests that the O.R. is a common arena for sexual references, as in the following joke told by an assisting O.R. doctor:

> Q: Do you know what happened to the nurse who swallowed a razor blade?
>
> A: She performed a tonsillectomy, a hysterectomy, and circumcised an intern.[34]

Yet while sexual references, images of fertility, and joking references to male and female bodies indicate renewal and rebirth, they also indicate that maleness is associated with medical competence and femaleness is associated with weakness, passivity, and failure. In *Scrubs*, Carla, the surgical intern's girlfriend, assists him as a nurse in the operating room. Once in the operating room she treats him as her partner, demanding, for example, that he say please and thank you when asking for surgical instruments. Carla explains to the other surgeons that she makes Turk (who is bald) wax his head. In response, the attending surgeon asks Turk, "Does she make you wax your vagina as well?" effectively feminizing Turk. In yet another episode, Dr. Cox writes J.D. a mock prescription.[35] The prescription, which is for "two testicles," is to be filled out immediately, implying that Dr. Dorian (J.D.) lacks maleness and, hence, competence as a doctor. In these examples, male doctors' bodies are "out of control," and they are told to obtain control by asserting masculinity.[36]

As carnivalesque laughter can simultaneously destroy and renew, it is inherently ambivalent, reaching its height of ambivalence with respect to death. At its most basic level, the totalizing nature of a modern hospital exists to control and contain death, which is in fact inevitable, unknowable, and uncontrollable. The absurd nature of this modern project is evident in the passage from *House of God* below, which graphically conflates humor, suffering, blood, death, and feces as manifested in a patient's uncontrollable body, which, however, is eventually saved:

> The nurse came in and said, "Mr. Lazarus has just had a bowel movement that is all blood."
>
> "Hey, that's really funny, Maxine. You got a great sense of humor."
>
> "No, I'm serious. The bed is solid blood."

> They wanted me to go on, and I could not. The world became the world just before the head-on crash. It could not be what it was. "I can't do anything more tonight," I heard myself say. "I'll see you in the morning."
> "Look, Roy, don't you understand? He's just bled out a gallon of blood. He's lying in it.
> You're the doctor, and you have to do something for him."
> Filled with hate, trying to get rid of thoughts that Lazarus wanted to die and I wanted him to die and I had to break my ass to stop him from dying, I went into his room and was face-to-face with black putrid sticky wet blood. On autopilot, I went to work.[37]

This example illustrates that, according to institutional scripts, doctors are supposed to stave off death at any cost, and some doctors consider it a personal failure when their patients die, even when they feel death is the "right" thing for the patient to do. On the other hand, doctors are more comfortable with death than the general population and a patient's immanent death often is a source of stress between doctors and patients' families. Families often want to prolong the patient's life as long as possible, while both the doctor and patient may consider it more humane to allow nature to take its course. At other times, it is the doctor who wants to prolong life more so than the patient and family. The medical carnivalesque performs this ambivalence through the extensive use of euphemisms and jokes about this inevitable finality of the human condition, laughing at the condition of human suffering and frailty and the futility of efforts to avoid death. In the following joke, for example, human suffering and sadness are rendered comical; death is the preferred outcome:

> A woman collapses in her home. Her son takes her to the hospital. The doctor returns and says to the son, "I have both good news and bad news."
>
> Son: Well, give me the bad news first.
>
> Doctor: Well, your mother has had a severe stroke and is completely incapacitated.
>
> You'll need to care for her every need for the rest of her life. You'll need to feed her, get her out of bed to go to the bathroom. You'll have to wipe her after she goes to the bathroom. You'll have to bathe her. She'll never speak again and she can't see or hear either. She can't walk, so you'll have to exercise her every day. Her nursing and medical needs will drain every penny you have. In fact, you'll be so stressed out from taking care of her, you will probably die first.
>
> Son: Oh my god. That's horrible. What's the good news?
>
> Doctor: HA! Just kidding. She's dead.

Further illustrating medical ambivalence toward death, there are a number of humorous terms for the elderly and other people who are about to die. An elderly patient who fails to thrive, for example, is said to be "dwindling," or has a case of the "dwindles." The dwindles stands for a series of health problems such as dementia, weight loss, inactivity, poor nutrition, depression, and others. Patients who are nearing death—such as one with a bad case of the dwindles—are said to be "circling the drain" or merely "lingering." In Britain, an elderly patient might be called a "wrinkly" or a "crumble"; s/he may also have a case of TMB (Too Many Birthdays) in which case, they may be sent to the "departure lounge" (geriatric ward).[38] The Brits may also call a patient T.F. BUNDY, which stands for Totally Fucked But Unfortunately Not Dead Yet, a term that conflates vulgar language, sexual references, and death.[39] Those who have died have gone to the ECU, or the "eternal care unit."[40]

Doctors perhaps are most ambivalent about those patients who don't improve but also don't die; the medical carnivalesque acknowledges the absurdity of trying to cure, heal, or otherwise "save" those patients who cannot be controlled. This ambivalence can be understood as the consequence of "creeping normalcy." Creeping normalcy refers to the acceptance of a major, otherwise intolerable, change as normal over time. After years of ongoing attempts to control the uncontrollable (in this case, death itself), physicians begin to accept these attempts as somehow normal. The incongruity resulting from creeping normalcy results in ambivalence.

From a doctor's perspective, the best possible situation is a patient who gets well and is discharged from the hospital. The patient is healthy and happy, and the doctor has less work to do. But there are some patients who not only cannot be discharged, but also don't seem to improve at all. In this case, the second best option is to move them to another doctor's service or onto another team. The terms "buffing" and "turfing" refer to ways in which this is accomplished. One "buffs" a patient—makes him/her look suitable for a different service—in order to "turf" them—move them out. These references to buffing present the patient's body as "polished" in order to look good—at least on the outside.

Some sick patients really do belong on one's service and are too sick to be discharged, remaining there for a long period of time. These patients are known as "rocks." The implication is that you can't move them, and that their state is unchangeable. Particularly obese patients who can't be moved are "boulders." Doctors with a lot of rocks on their service are known as "rock collectors," or as having "rock gardens." "How's the rock garden?" is a question these caregivers endure.

The most well-known patient-type who cannot be discharged is the "gomer." The term "gomer" refers to an elderly male patient, often a veteran, who never dies but also who never seems to leave the hospital. George and Dundes point out that this is the patient from whom one cannot escape and therefore is one of the most uncontrollable kind of patients that exist. In the 1970s, the classic gomer figure was unkempt, missing teeth, alcoholic, and dirty[41]; today the term refers to a debilitated, elderly, senile patient who cannot be healed.[42] In *Scrubs* gomers are described as old people "who don't have the decency to die," while the term "Gomer Pile" refers to the care unit for these chronically sick patients.[43] In *The House of God*, Gomer is also an acronym for Get Out of My E.R.,[44] suggesting that the patient is wasting the doctor's time, an idea illustrated by the following discussion between Fats and Potts.

> Potts: "I've got some work to do."
>
> Fats: "Well, you won't believe this either, but most of the work you do doesn't matter. For the care of these gomers, it doesn't matter a damn."[45]

George and Dundes also found the term "grume" in use at the time of their article, "The Gomer: A Figure of American Hospital Folk Speech." A grume is worse than a gomer and refers to a blood clot or a pile of feces.[46] A female gomer may be called a gomere, or she may simply be a LOL in NAD (Little Old Lady in No Apparent Distress).[47]

Gomers are identified by exaggerated, debased physical characteristics and their ability to evade hospital release. In one of several "Gomer Assessment Sheets" collected, points are assigned to assess gomerdom. If a patient has been unemployed since World War II for lower back pain, for instance, he (gomers are mostly male) is assigned three points; if he has been unemployed for lower back pain since the Spanish American War, he is assigned fifteen points. A patient wins ten points if he urinates on a physician, twelve points for drinking from a urinal, and four points for biting the bulb off a rectal thermometer.[48]

Derisive, carnivalesque laughter is the best way to deal with such uncontrollable patients. In *The House of God*, Dr. Basch narrates, "A shriek came from the gomere: REEE-REEE-REEEEE . . . and all I did, while they stared at me, was lie on the tile floor and laugh. . . . these gomers had won."[49] Early in Dr. Basch's training, he quickly discovers the sad state of these patients:

> When I [Dr. Basch], laughing, told her [Berry, his girlfriend] about Harry the Horse and the farting Jane Doe, she didn't laugh. "How can you laugh at that? They sound pathetic." "They are. . . ."[50]

According to Dr. Basch, gomers are not only pathetic, they are absurd; and as living absurdities, they embody the futility of the modern medical project and thus deserve mockery and scorn. *Scrubs* illustrates gomer status by one patient's inability to say anything but the word "pickles." The episode opens with J.D. heaping mocking abuse on the patient. J.D. asks the gomer a series of questions, to which the patient responds "pickles." J.D. finally asks him "Peter Piper picked a peck of pickled—what?" When the gomer responds "pickles," J.D. mocks him saying "*NO*, the correct answer is *pepper*. Peter Piper picked a peck of pickled *peppers*." Comic praise and abuse are two sides of the same coin. Upon discovering J.D. ridiculing the patient, Dr. Cox praises him, saying, "God, I've never felt closer to you before." Here, the praise issued by Dr. Cox allows the caregivers to acknowledge mutually the futility of their efforts and to agree that mockery is the appropriate response.

In *Rabelais*, abuse occurs in a variety of forms, including verbal invectives as well as actual physical beatings, which Bakhtin understood as a means of revival and regeneration. While symbolic abuse may not necessarily be a form of renewal in the medical carnivalesque, it occurs frequently enough to warrant notice:

> Potts' head turned to watch the Fat Man go, and somehow, her left hand free, Ina slugged him again. Reflexively Potts raised his hand to hit her, and then stopped himself. The Fat Man nearly keeled over with laughter. "Ho ho, did you see that? I love 'em, I love these gomers, I do...." And he laughed his way out the door.[51]

Comic abuse not only occurs with patients but between doctors. In one episode of *Scrubs*, Dr. Cox punches Dr. Kelso in the nose and follows this show of aggression with a verbal attack of a sexual nature: "That felt so good I changed my pants afterwards." The rest of the episode revolves around the comical result of the punch, which is that Dr. Kelso's nose squeaks as he breathes.

Comic abuse and debasement occur in jokes and slang as well, as in the following example:

> Q: What's the difference between a pile of shit and an intern [or medical student]?
> A: You don't go out of your way to step on a pile of shit.[52]

The acronym BOHICA, which stands for Bend Over Here It Comes Again, conflates abuse with anal sex.[53] While of course no doctor would tolerate the actual abuse of patients or colleagues, humor is used as an effective tool to establish or remind those entrenched in the medical community about dominance, power, hierarchy, and roles. No one person or position is beyond reproach.

## CONCLUSION

Western biomedicine both embodies and drives modern understandings of life, health, and death, and it does so through technologies of the body. According to biomedical ideologies, death is understood as existing in opposition to life, the result of life's failure rather than its culmination or end result. Beliefs of "death as the enemy" and "death as a failure" pervade the medical community, indicating a shift from the notion that death is a part of life to the idea that death can be avoided or indefinitely delayed.[54] The idea that death can be avoided illustrates the powerful influence of creeping normalcy inherent in current medical culture and society in general:

> Youth is celebrated as the ideal; longevity is desired, and remains a primary standard for evaluating health-care systems; and when a friend or relative is dying people commonly avoid the person, feeling that "I don't know what to do or say." The focus has been on avoiding problems and stopping bad interventions rather than on a positive ideal of a good death.[54]

As instantiated in hospital settings, the biomedical project ultimately wields power over death by offering a rationalization of it. Since death cannot be avoided completely, the goal becomes commanding, containing, and controlling it. In pursuit of this goal, human bodies are analyzed, manipulated, managed, and mastered through technology and medicine, resulting in surreal and often ridiculous situations. If medicine has at times been likened to a theater, these situations reveal its occasional absurd nature.

The medical carnivalesque acknowledges the irrationality deeply rooted in this very modern project. Drawing upon the grotesque out-of-control body as a traditional symbolic resource, the medical carnivalesque conflates excrement, sex, disease, disability, and death to mock and deride human attempts to control life and death. In doing so, the medical carnivalesque challenges biomedical ideologies of control by turning them on their ear and rolling them on their bellies. If the hospital is a rationalized institution, the medical carnivalesque points out the cracks in its foundations. If patients are sacrosanct, the medical carnivalesque points out the futility of their battle to prolong life or stave off death. If medical trainees are managers, the medical carnivalesque shows them as barkers in a three-ring circus. If the attending physicians are performers, the medical carnivalesque flaunts them as ring masters. No part of the institution is immune to its laughter.

Following Bakhtin, we suggest that the medical carnivalesque does not merely mock or degrade but also renews. Carnivalesque laughter is regenerative, offering a way out of impossible situations, at least on the symbolic level. While previous scholars have acknowledged the importance of humor in medical settings to cope with highly chaotic and stressful situations, the nature of its ambivalence has escaped theorization. Doctors often are ambivalent about their work, and this ambivalence emerges in humor. One can attempt to control and rationalize death, but death refuses rationalization, and if one cannot laugh at these attempts, then one must cry.

In bringing together life and death within a single unified symbolic framework, the medical carnivalesque accomplishes deeply serious and important work. The ability to symbolize humorously what medical professionals do as absurd requires an awareness of their own human frailty and powerlessness. The biomedical model, which reduces caregivers to mere technicians, dehumanizes not only patients but also those who would heal. Those who can't laugh, who take themselves too seriously and perceive what they do as "normal," are the ones who are lost. In *Labyrinth of Solitude*, Octavio Paz famously noted the ability of the Mexican people to face death through laughter. While the idea of laughing at death now has become a cliché of the Mexican national character, the practice still holds sway in other arenas.[56] As Narváez concludes, "the commingling of humor and death in informal and ritualistic circumstances appears to be a human universal, a technique for communicating and dealing with the enigma of our precarious mortality."[57] It is by laughing at human suffering, disease, and failure that the fear of death, if not death itself, is conquered. As the Irish proverb says, A good laugh and a long sleep are the best cures in the doctor's book.

## NOTES

1. Michel Foucault, *The Birth of the Clinic: An Archaeology of Medical Perception* (New York: Vintage Books, [1973]1994).

2. The term "totalizing institution" refers to institutions where the normal activities of a group of people are determined and regulated within a designated space for the purpose of achieving an overarching goal. See Erving Goffman, *Asylums: Essays on the Social Situation of Mental Patients and Other Inmates* (Garden City, NY: Anchor-Doubleday 1961).

3. Robyn Wiegman, *American Anatomies: Theorizing Race and Gender* (Durham: Duke University Press, 1995).

4. Jay Mechling, "Children's Folklore in Residential Institutions: Summer Camps, Boarding Schools, Hospitals and Custodial Facilities," in *Children's Folklore: A Sourcebook*, ed. Brian Sutton-Smith, Jay Mechling, Thomas W. Johnson, and Felicia R. McMahon (Logan: Utah State University Press, 1999), 273–91.

5. Victoria George and Alan Dundes, "The Gomer: A Figure of American Hospital Folk Speech," *Journal of American Folklore* 91, no. 359 (1978): 568–81; Anne Burson-Tolpin, "Fracturing the Language of Biomedicine: The Speech Play of U.S. Physicians," *Medical Anthropology Quarterly* New Series 3, no. 4 (1989): 283–93; Jamie Moore, "Poetry, Puns, and Pediatrics: The Verbal Artistry of Dr. James L. Hughes," *North Carolina Folklore Journal* 38, no. 1 (1991): 45–71; Kathleen Odean, "Anal Folklore in the Medical World," in *Folklore Interpreted: Essays in Honor of Alan Dundes*, ed. Regina Bendix and Rosemary Lévy Zumwalt (New York and London: Garland Publishing, Inc., 1995), 137–52; Paul Grayson, "The Folklore of a Medical Community," *Louisiana Folklore Miscellany* 5 (1981): 48–52; Yvette Trahant, "The Oral Tradition of the Physician," *Louisiana Folklore Miscellany* 5 (1981): 38–47; Rose Laub Coser, "Some Social Functions of Laughter: A Study of Humor in a Hospital Setting," *Human Relations* 12 (1959):171–82; Robert H. Coombs, Sangeeta Chopra, Debra R. Schenk, and Elaine Yutan, "Medical Slang and Its Functions," *Social Science and Medicine* 36, no. 8 (1993): 987–998; Adam T. Fox, Michael Fertleman, Pauline Cahill, and Roger D. Palmer, "Medical Slang in British Hospitals," *Ethics and Behavior* 13, no. 2 (2003):173–89; Vera M. Robinson, *Humor and the Health Professions* (Thorofare, NJ: Charles B. Slack, Inc., 1977).

6. Genevieve Noone Parsons, Sara B. Kinsman, Charles L. Bosk, Pamela Sankar, and Peter A. Ubel, "Between Two Worlds: Medical Student Perceptions of Humor and Slang in the Hospital Setting," *Journal of General Internal Medicine* 16 (2001): 544–49; Frederic W. Hafferty, "Cadaver Stories and the Emotional Socialization of Medical Students," *Journal of Health and Social Behavior* 29, no. 4 (1988): 344–56.

7. Peter Narváez, ed. *Of Corpse: Death and Humor in Folklore and Popular Culture* (Logan: Utah State University Press, 2003), 5ff.

8. Mikhail Bakhtin, *Rabelais and His World*, trans. Hélène Iswolsky (Bloomington: Indiana University Press, 1984).

9. George L. Engel, "The Need for a New Medical Model: A Challenge for Biomedicine," *Science* 196, no. 4286 (1977): pp. 129–36, 131.

10. Ibid., 131.

11. Anthony Giddens, *The Consequences of Modernity* (Stanford: Stanford University Press, 1990), 83ff.

12. Arthur Kleinman, *The Illness Narratives: Suffering, Healing and the Human Condition* (New York: Basic Books, Inc., 1988), 5-6.

13. Arthur W. Frank, *The Wounded Storyteller: Body, Illness, and Ethics* (Chicago: University of Chicago Press, 1995), 66.

14. Felice Aull and Bradley Lewis, "Medical Intellectuals: Resisting Medical Orientalism," *Journal of the Medical Humanities* 25, no. 2 (2004):87-108; Renee R. Anspach, "Notes on the Sociology of Medical Discourse: The Language of Case Presentation," *Journal of Health and Social Behavior* 29, no. 4 (1988): 357-75; William J. Donnelly, "The Language of Medical Case Histories," *Annals of Internal Medicine* 127, no. 11 (December, 1997): 1045-48.

15. Frank, *The Wounded Storyteller*, 34.

16. Eric J. Cassell, "The Nature of Suffering and the Goals of Medicine," *New England Journal of Medicine* 306, no. 11 (1982): 640.

17. Samuel Shem, *The House of God: The Classic Novel of Life and Death in an American Hospital* (New York: Random House, Inc., [1978]2003), 47.

18. Bakhtin, *Rabelais and His World*, 317.

19. Ibid., 370ff.

20. Mahadev L. Apte, "Humor," in *Folklore, Cultural Performances, and Popular Entertainments*, ed. Richard Bauman (Oxford: Oxford University Press, 1992), 67-75, 68.

21. Bakhtin, *Rabelais and His World*, 147.

22. Odean's "Anal Folklore in the Medical World" was published appropriately as a *festschrift* for folklorist Alan Dundes, who (in)famously was interested in such matters from a Freudian perspective.

23. Odean, "Anal Folklore in the Medical World," 139.

24. Ibid., 142.

25. Ibid., 145.

26. Coombs et al., "Medical Slang and Its Functions," 990.

27. Odean, "Anal Folklore in the Medical World," 142.

28. Robinson, *Humor and the Health Professions*, 70.

29. Bakhtin, *Rabelais and His World*, 192-93.

30. Shem, *The House of God*, 33.

31. Odean, "Anal Folklore in the Medical World," 138.

32. Fox et al., "Medical Slang in British Hospitals," 188.

33. Shem, *The House of God*, 164-69.

34. Robinson, *Humor and the Health Professions*, 70.

35. Bakhtin associates mock prescriptions with the laughter of the quack and druggest at the fair, *Rabelais and His World*, 185–87.

36. Jeannie B. Thomas discusses women's resourceful use of Bakhtinian laughter as it emerges in personal experience narratives and life histories in her book *Featherless Chickens, Laughing Women, and Serious Stories* (Charlottesville: University Press of Virginia, 1997). See particularly her chapter entitled "Laughter, Ambivalence and the Body," pp. 73–128.

37. Shem, *The House of God*, 121–22.

38. Fox et al., "Medical Slang in British Hospitals," 183, 89.

39. Ibid., 188.

40. George and Dundes, "The Gomer," 569.

41. Ibid., 570.

42. Deborah B. Leiderman and Jean-Anne Grisso, "The Gomer Phenomenon," *Journal of Health and Social Behavior* 26, no. 3 (1985): pp. 222–32, p. 225.

43. Coombs et al., "Medical Slang and Its Functions," 989.

44. Shem, *The House of God*, 29.

45. Ibid., 44.

46. George and Dundes, "The Gomer," 572.

47. Shem, *The House of God*, 33.

48. George and Dundes, "The Gomer," 575–79.

49. Shem, *The House of God*, 286.

50. Ibid., 24.

51. Ibid., 36.

52. Odean, "Anal Folklore in the Medical World," 145.

53. Ibid., 146.

54. Ira Byock writes specifically: "As a clinician it seems disrespectful to discuss the 'meaning and value' of death. The preciousness of life underlies all clinical disciplines and preservation of life is a paramount clinical goal. Understandably, for clinicians death is the enemy to be conquered, and when it occurs, it represents defeat and failure." Ira Byock, "The Meaning and Value of Death," *Journal of Palliative Medicine* 5, no. 2 (2002): 279–88, p. 279. Howard Brody writes about medicine's fascination with and belief in rescue: "The rescue fantasy is a power trip: it envisions the physician having the power to snatch the patient from the jaws of death." See Howard Brody, *The Healer's Power* (New Haven: Yale University Press, 1992), 139.

55. Ezekiel J. Emanuel and Linda L. Emanuel, "The Promise of a Good Death," *Lancet* 351, supplement II (1998): 5II 21–29, p. 21.

56. Stanley Brandes, "Is There a Mexican View of Death?" *Ethos* 31, no. 1 (2003): 127–44.

57. Narváez, 11.

ELEVEN

# Dr. Jarvik and Other Baby Boomers

## (Still) Performing the Able Body

========

LINDA SEIDEL

we tend to fear old age as
some sort of disorder   that can be cured
with the proper brand of aspirin
or perhaps a bit of Ben Gay for the shoulders
it does   of course   pay to advertise.
　　　　　　　　　　　　—Nikki Giovanni, "Age"

Each of us has a disabled other who cannot be acknowledged.
　　　　　　　　　　　　—Henri-Jacques Stiker

IN A COMMERCIAL YOU MIGHT see on the evening news, an aging Dr. Robert
Jarvik, path-breaking inventor of the artificial heart, rows a gleaming sports
kayak across a gorgeous mountain-rimmed lake. The camera moves back
and forth between Jarvik's demonstration of physical fitness and the
doctor's advice to the viewer about the value of Lipitor in helping to maintain heart health. The doctor's hair is thinning and gray, but he can row
fast. (We never learn whether *he* takes Lipitor or not.) In another ad targeted at the news-watching middle-aged, two fifty-something husbands (one
white, white black), with wives hovering nearby, sing the praises of Levitra
for reversing their erectile dysfunction. In a Fosamax commercial, a succes-
sion of "doctors" (actors wearing lab coats and stethoscopes) of various

races, ages, and genders seem to address "you," their patient, directly, explaining how their pill will rebuild the bone you have lost due to "post-menopausal osteoporosis" and prevent potentially lethal fractures.

As these examples illustrate, prescription drug commercials targeted at a middle-aged and older audience play upon ableist and ageist fears that we will lose our sexual potency, our grace, and our very ability to function *normally* in a society where normal functioning is keyed to young able-bodied-ness. Thus, the ordinary slowing of sexual response as one ages becomes medicalized as a condition to be treated. The decline in athleticism that even the physically fit are liable to experience as they grow older is to be staved off as long as possible through the use of the correct pill, lest they have to admit the advance of age or disability. (Ironically, the pill in question may not directly enhance one's able-bodiedness at all, but the commercial implies that it does, as in the case of the Lipitor ad.)

In this chapter, I will argue that current advertising reinforces the stigmas associated with age and disability as they are written on the body and reinscribes the perfect young, able body as everyone's unattainable ideal. At the same time, even as the ads coerce us to remain able-bodied according to market-induced standards, they show us that we have plenty of company in not meeting those standards at all. Whether we have to urinate too often, need to monitor our diabetes, can't become erect, or no longer move with the agility of youth, we now know that we have plenty of company. All those people in the ads tell us so.

## COMPULSORY ABLE-BODIEDNESS

Yet the impact of prescription drug ads on viewers as a source of information (however misleading) and attitude creation is relatively recent. It was only in 1997 that the FDA removed the requirement that advertisements include a "brief summary" of all drug side effects, "clearing the way for an avalanche of new pharma TV ads."[1] While the pharmaceutical companies (or "pharma") spent $2 million on direct-to-consumer (DTC) advertising in 1980, by 2004 the figure had risen to $4.35 billion (Critser 6). As a result, drug use in the United States is way up despite the substantial health risks and the huge financial costs, because, as Greg Critser argues in *Generation Rx*, we have allowed big pharma to change our culture sufficiently that we now think we need the performance enhancement and prolongation of youth promised by the ads (2-9).

Some of us are seduced by the testimony of celebrities, who praise the enhancement of their lives by the drug they are well paid to sell.[2] For example, in a commercial current several years ago, Dorothy Hamill glides across the ice, her middle-aged body showing no signs of the arthritis that threatens to disable her, she claims, should she fail to take the high-priced anti-inflammatory Vioxx (pulled from the market in October 2004 because it was implicated in thousands of heart attacks). Although I was never tempted to take Vioxx myself, I was fascinated: Here was a beautiful, still-vigorous athlete admitting her vulnerability! Perhaps I identified more, though, with the grandmotherly black woman who took Vioxx to keep up with the children in the elementary school class she taught: She just wanted to be able to do her job. The fact that there are now many thousands of lawsuits pending against Merck by the alleged victims of Vioxx and their families suggests that DTC advertising drives up consumer expectations with respect to the able functioning of the aging body without necessarily being able to fulfill them.

As a baby boomer myself, I feel that I too am in danger of being seduced. If you count the cholesterol pill I have been persuaded to take, maybe I have lost my pharmaceutical virginity already. I am a member of the generation that is supposed to break the national bank when we get *really* old. In my current incarnation, my left knee hurts after too much dancing and my back gets stiff. Lest I imagine that I will deteriorate no further, I have the examples of my parents' cases to suggest otherwise. My eighty-six-year-old mother cannot walk without assistance; my eighty-one-year-old father is in the early stages of Alzheimer's. Now it's true that I never did have the perfectly able body: My eyes have always been near-sighted and astigmatic; I was the slowest runner in my gym class; I dropped more food items than any other server when I tried to work as a waitress during my college years. Still, my feelings of insecurity about the possible future loss of my modest physical powers are relatively new. I am ripe for exploitation, or so the commercial advertisements targeted toward my age group seem to suggest. And, although I have not felt moved to buy any of the expensive prescription drugs that are supposed to maintain the smooth functioning of my muscles or enhance my waning sexual desire or still the contractions of an overactive bladder, I nonetheless take these commercials personally. I know they mean me.

Marxist philosopher Louis Althusser gives me the language by which I can explain my experience. Although he was writing before the era of DTC drug advertising, he described similar ideological come-ons as methods by which capitalist regimes might reproduce themselves. He wrote that "ideology... 'recruits' subjects among the individuals... or 'transforms' the individuals into subjects" by the process of "*interpellation* or hailing... which can be imagined along the lines of the most commonplace everyday police (or other) hailing: 'Hey, you there!'"[3] Thus, prescription drug ads interpellate viewers according to the audience being targeted. *I am interpellated by* ads that seem to say: "Hey, you aging boomer who is becoming, or might become, disabled soon. Hey, you don't have the right to become that disabled person when you can avoid that fate by taking our pill." And the come-on asks us to *become* the person to whom the pill can be sold—that person for whom normality means functioning like our young, able-bodied self, but also that person who can already see or fear middle-aged and elderly deterioration. The commercials are powerful because they do not simply say, "You need this product." Rather, they say, "You *are* this potentially disabled person, yet you cannot afford to be. *You* are the one we made these pills for."

The process of interpellation is not complete, however, until "the hailed individual...turn[s] around": "By this mere one-hundred-and-eighty-degree physical conversion, he becomes a *subject*. Why? Because he has recognized that the hail was 'really' addressed to him...(and not someone else)" (Althusser 174). If the mirror (which reflects back to us social expectations as well as our own image) or the reactions of others (another kind of mirror) are not enough to convince us of our incipient decrepitude, the prescription drug ads invite us to say, "Oh, *I am* that person who must try to stay fit—for my family, my students, my co-workers, my sense of myself as strong and independent." Viewers of drug ads, as Althusser would predict, typically accept the ideological premises on which they are predicated, and those premises are reinforced by viewing the ad. They include the need for autonomy and able-bodiedness and the compulsion to try to perform as one did in youth. If, as Lennard Davis says, disability is "located in the observer,"[4] then the ads trying to sell us Celebrex, Cialis, and so forth, invite us to observe *ourselves* as potentially, incipiently, or already disabled *unless* we take the pills. The ads won't work unless we identify with their protagonists who fight to retain their normality.

Robert McRuer, in his discussion of "compulsory able-bodiedness," points out that able-bodiedness is an ideal none of us can ever really *achieve*; rather, we can approximate it for awhile if we are lucky. But it's always a performance (much as gender is a performance, according to Judith Butler), and, as we grow older, the performance is bound to deviate from the cultural standards set out for us as compulsory.[5] Thus, the drugs targeted for the aging body could, in a very real sense, be described as *performance-enhancing*—not just in a sexual sense, but enhancing of the consumer's capacity to perform continuing able-bodiedness convincingly.

In sketching the development of the able-bodied ideal, McRuer connects "the compulsory nature of able-bodiedness" with the nineteenth-century "rise of industrial capitalism" and the demand for workers "capable of the normal physical exertions required in a particular system of labor" (McRuer 91-92). Davis similarly argues that in the "industrial-political notion of democracy" that arose in the nineteenth century, workers were thought of as "interchangeable.... Clearly people with disabilities pose problems to work situations in which labor is standardized and bodies conceptualized as interchangeable."[6] According to Critser, the demands of the workplace are now helping to drive the marketing and consumption of expensive prescription drugs: "Almost all chronic-disease drugs are sold because they increase performance, sustain productivity, lessen pain, or increase longevity. They are all...drugs for a work-based culture" (137). Disabilities (including those perceived to be incipient), then, are defined by the demands of the workplace, but, ironically, those demands for "ever increasing productivity" have become a "source of modern illness" (Critser 139). Yet the medical model of problem-solving, exploited by pharma, tends to ignore environmental and institutional causes of distress in favor of treating discrete individuals for their presumably individual problems (Critser 145).

Of course, prescription drugs are not the only products that help us fit in at work. As Harlan Hahn, in "Advertising the Acceptably Employable Image," notes, we are expected to "transform" ourselves by using products that supposedly bring us closer to accepted cultural norms.[7] Surely we all understand, even as we are loath to admit, that commercials play a huge role in determining what we think bodies should be or do (Hahn 176–80). Deodorant ads may not persuade us to buy any particular product, for example, but they help create the expectation that human bodies are not allowed to have ordinary human animal odors, and if we do have them, we must get rid of them as quickly as possible. This has become an irreversible bourgeois expectation, so that one risks social shunning and workplace repercussions if one dares to exude one's own natural odors.

Similarly, we are not supposed to "give in" to arthritis pain when there are pills we can take to make us just as active and reliable as our families and workplaces want us to be. We may be asked to take the pill for ourselves, for our own benefit, but if that isn't enough, we are reminded to do it for others—for those who need our labor or our care, or for those who simply don't want us burdening them. Thus, the grandmotherly-looking black woman in the Vioxx commercial can brag that she can keep up with the young schoolchildren in her classroom and that her students hardly ever have a substitute. (What will she do now that Vioxx has been taken off the market because it causes heart trouble? Switch to another high-priced drug? Rethink her priorities? But the latter course would reject the "fight" we all are supposed to engage in to overcome real or incipient impairments.)

The plot of the prescription pill commercial typically follows what Paul Darke calls "the normality drama."[8] Writing about "cinematic representations of disability," Darke notes the supremacy of the medical model in which "impairment" is presented "as an individual, pathological, problem to be either overcome or eradicated" (181, 184). Many commercials are normality dramas in miniature with an impaired protagonist who gets "cured" or whose impairment is ameliorated or alleviated to the point of being invisible. We are shown the person in her or his "abnormal" mode (she has to pee too often; he can't get it up) and then in the triumphal mode produced by the drug being advertised. Or we skip right to the triumphal mode, in which the earlier impairment (not being able to walk without pain, say) is just a memory that enhances the present pleasure.

The commercials are "nostalgic" (Darke 194) in that the aging protagonist regains the powers of youth. S/he is not allowed to slow down or grow old gracefully because school children demand an active teacher, fans can recognize only a Dorothy Hamill who skates, and lovers supposedly desire virile partners. But I suspect that it is not only this relentless external pressure to perform that haunts us: Would Dorothy Hamill be able to recognize *herself* if she could not skate? And if she suspects she could not, then the compulsion to take the rejuvenating pill, despite the possible side effects, is very strong.

Of course, the commercials suggest our fragility even as they promise cure or amelioration because the aging body is multiply vulnerable in the sense of falling away from the standards of youth. You fix one thing (arthritis, say) only to find that you have high cholesterol or a hearing loss or a sexual dysfunction—so we are "fighting" a losing battle, if the goal is to regain the youthful, "able-bodied" self (which was never perfectly able-bodied to begin with). Yet the commercials appeal, in Lennard Davis's words, to that "imperative...to fit in," to be normal, and we are vulnerable to the appeal (*BB* 105). To ignore it is to risk being considered freakish or burdensome or, merely, old.

Davis argues that we have "the right to be ill, to be infirm, to be impaired without suffering discrimination or oppression" (*BB*, 1). That is, we have the right to refuse treatment that would render us less noticeably infirm, but which might cost too much in other ways: nasty side effects, exorbitant financial burdens, or the sense that our pills are making us less or other than ourselves. Davis observes that we avoid the subject of disability because we are all afraid we are headed there and notes that "It isn't necessarily bad to be disabled, but it is bad to be discriminated against" (*BB* 4-5). According to Davis, "disability is itself an unstable category" (*BB* 23), which makes me wonder whether today's commercials will succeed in raising the bar so high that last year's normal aging will become tomorrow's disability? Davis argues that capitalist pressures to maintain the "consumer-designed body" have very little to do with "caring *about* the body," which we, typically, do not do: Witness the existence of landmines, sweatshops, clitorectomies, and many other bodily abuses here and abroad (*BB* 27, 29).

## COMPULSORY NORMALITY

Given that the idea of normality is less than two hundred years old, there is nothing necessary or eternal about it (Davis, *BB* 105). Previously, there had been a conception of the *ideal,* which meant a standard too high for ordinary people to meet—which means that they did not *have* to meet it (Davis, *BB* 105). Davis traces the rise of the regime of the normal to "the development of statistics and of the bell curve, called...the 'normal' curve" in the early years of the nineteenth century. To begin with, then, norms were the products of statistical averages, supposedly describing what most people already were. Yet this paradigm shift meant new pressure on the outliers, the "abnormal," to fit in and conform to the norms that most other people already met (Davis, *BB* 105).

This tension between norms as descriptive averages and norms as prescriptive standards is very much present in contemporary medicine, at least where the use of drugs is concerned. To be more precise, averages obtained by measuring the blood pressure or bone density (for examples) of young healthy people may become the new standards everyone is supposed to meet. Moynihan and Cassels report that a World Health Organization study group "decided that 'normal' bone density was [that] of a young woman (a thirty-year-old)—a definition that automatically made the bones of many older women 'abnormal'" (Moynihan and Cassels 142).

That medical norms are not just averages anymore, but have moved in the direction of absolute standards, can be illustrated by a recent conversation between my family doctor and me. He twitted me with the fact that my blood pressure was 140 over 75 instead of 130 over 75, as usual. "It must have been those salty crab cakes I had for lunch," I hypothesized, refusing to be concerned. Perhaps to make peace, he responded by talking about a Paul Harvey radio show he had heard in which that opinionated commentator had argued that old people should be able to have the average blood pressure for an old person without being considered abnormal (and therefore in need of medication)—even though those numbers would be higher than the currently accepted standards. My doctor seemed faintly scandalized by this view. Yet Moynihan and Cassels cite experts who claim that hypertension, by itself, may not greatly increase the risk of heart attacks in otherwise healthy people (91).

Where the "normal" standards are set, of course, not only helps determine who can be urged to consume prescription drugs (often at substantial expense and some risk to themselves), but it also helps to establish *behavioral* norms for the responsible middle-aged or elderly person. Since we do not enjoy "the right to be ill, to be infirm, to be impaired without suffering discrimination or oppression" (Davis, *BB* 1), we dutifully take our pills, lest we should be blamed for whatever maladies do befall us. Yet "impairment is the rule, and normalcy is the fantasy," according to Davis, who therefore wants "a shift from the ideology of normalcy... to a vision of the body as changeable, imperfectable, unruly, and untidy" (Davis, *BB* 31, 39).

Rosemarie Garland-Thomson moves us closer to this vision in her book *Extraordinary Bodies*. Garland-Thomson pairs "the disabled figure" with "the normate" (her coinage), "the figure outlined by the array of deviant others whose marked bodies shore up the normate's boundaries."[9] This "constructed identity" allows its possessor to "step into [and maintain] a position of authority" (Garland-Thomson 8). Normates get to be authority figures, in part because their bodies can be ignored. That is, they seem to have no bodies at all, and the "disembodied" mind remains the literally impossible norm in a culture that still divides mind from body and still assigns bodies to those of lower status. Moreover, lower-status people are not just embodied, but trapped in bodies we cannot forget because, perhaps, they menstruate or give birth or get sick or age or exhibit a skin tone other than white. Embodiment itself, then, becomes a kind of deviance whose embarrassments we are constantly trying to escape. Thus, in the mind-body dichotomy, the self is lined up with the mind, and the body is supposed to cooperate or, at least, stay out of the way.

Commercials for prescription pills marketed to the middle-aged and elderly, then, play to some idealized notion of *who we really are* (as dictated by fantasies, cultural ideals, memories of one's capacities in youth, or envy of the apparently superior capacities of friends, siblings, and role models). The ads claim that the right pill will help us recapture the abilities of youth or achieve heights of virility or passion never experienced before. The promise of the pills is not just to relieve pain or enhance performance; it is to allow us to continue to define ourselves in particular ways or even to encourage the fantasy of a new, improved self-definition (see Garland-Thomson 47).

Because the prescription drug advertisements count on the continuing regime of compulsory able-bodiedness to help them sell their products, they are in the business of modeling, for older people, how to remain able-bodied, not how to be disabled. In fact, there are very few representations of how to be disabled—of how one might usefully think of oneself and negotiate the world as a disabled person. Garland-Thomson argues that "[t]he discursive construct of the disabled figure" is "informed more by received attitudes than by people's actual experience of disability," which is infrequently and inadequately represented. Moreover, "received attitudes" are reflected, created, and maintained in powerful works of literature, where the disabled person is made to represent a variety of spiritual maladies as well as the body's own fragility (Garland-Thomson 9-15). Thus, Ahab in *Moby Dick* is tragic because he has lost the power of self-definition: He "is not a self-made man, but a whale-made man; his disabled body testifies to the self's physical vulnerability, the ominous knowledge that the ideology of individualism suppresses" (Garland-Thomson 45).

## A DIFFERENT BODY

No tragic figures, of course, appear in prescription drug ads, just the "compliant bod[ies]" required "to secure a place in the fiercely competitive and dynamic socioeconomic realm" (Garland-Thomson 43). Our jobs, our love lives, and our very selves are at stake, it would seem, should we cease to remain fit. And yet Americans are, possibly, the most unfit people in the world. We eat too much, exercise too little, and expect quick fixes from pills and plastic surgery. Without making a defense of obesity, which I do see as a public health problem brought to us by the same capitalist system that sells us pills, I would like to suggest that the time may have come for us to accept—perhaps celebrate—a diversity of body types and capabilities. Building on the work of queer theorist Michael Warner, who argues that everyone is "virtually queer" and that some of us choose to be "critically queer" as well,[10] Robert McRuer notes that all of us are "virtually disabled": If we are able-bodied, we are temporarily so, and we can never fulfill the norms of perfect able-bodiedness in any case (95-96). McRuer, then, invites us to take deliberately "a critically disabled position": one that is critical of the regime of compulsory able-bodiedness and unashamedly nonassimilationist (96). In *The Trouble with Normal*, Warner shows that the ordinary way of fighting the stigma of abnormality, which is to change the standards of what is considered normal, leaves the normal vs. abnormal hierarchy intact.[11] Warner, McRuer, Davis, Garland-Thomson, and others argue for the acceptance of differences without hierarchizing them.

Never having felt all that normal myself, I find the rejection of the whole regime of the normal an attractive idea. But, since the concept of normality is such a powerful social tool—and possibly not all bad (Would we have more crime without it? Or would we simply reduce our sky-high incarceration rate?)—it seems unlikely that we will jettison "normality" any time soon. Yet as the baby boomers age, it does seem likely that this term will be stretched and challenged in new ways. Some of us will, undoubtedly, take the pills and the tummy tucks in the attempt to hold onto a youthful version of ourselves, including an able-bodied presentation, as long as possible. Others of us, I hope, will insist upon our right to be regarded as fully human even as we cling to our walkers, propel ourselves in wheelchairs, or acknowledge that our memories aren't what they used to be.

The medical experts and the media pundits talk about the aging of my generation as a potential health catastrophe and a financial burden on younger people (the people who seem to count). But I want to see our collective aging as an opportunity to rethink old age, to reclaim the adjective "old" as descriptive rather than pejorative, to make it cool to be old. I want the protestors of the 1960s to claim our rights as the octogenarians of the 2020s. When medication helps us pursue that project, we must demand it for ourselves. But when medication simply renders us more manageable by others, more compliant, more "normal," we have the responsibility to insist that normalization of our aging bodies may not be our number-one goal or even an outcome to be desired.

Becoming knowledgeable consumers, however, is no easy task—especially because our chief source of information about prescription drugs is advertising, and drug companies do their best to minimize our legitimate skepticism and promote themselves as working hard solely for the benefit of humankind. Just in case the Vioxx scandals have disillusioned us, pharma runs public relations ads about its high standards of ethics, its devotion to the public good, and the touching success stories it has already made possible or which, it predicts, are just around the corner. It promises to *take care* of us. Astra Zeneca, for example, invites prospective patients to contact the company for financial aid if they cannot afford the medications. Yet, according to Critser, "pharma's principal allegiances are not to God, nature, and men, but to science, markets, and mammon" (253).

Drug ads, justified by pharma as simply informational, not only promote awareness of particular drugs but also of the sometimes newly created conditions they are supposed to treat. The development of Pfizer's Viagra is an interesting case in point. Critser reports that Viagra was "originally tested for treatment of angina," was proved ineffective, but was shown to produce erections as a side effect. Soon Pfizer went looking for a "'disease' that regarded an erection as a 'cure.' The answer was a condition dubbed 'erectile dysfunction,' or ED" (95). The rest, as they say, is history. (Curiously, it is the young, already potent, who have become more enamored of Viagra than the elderly [Critser 95], perhaps an indication that the elderly really are more mature!)

Yet, as misleading and biased as drug advertising can be, it may be the *only* source of information readily available to many people. For example, I was not told by my doctor about the possible side effects of the choles-terol-reducing drug I take; I heard about them on TV. Thus, I am of two minds about the advertising of prescription drugs to middle-aged and older people.

If the advertisements, in part, create the impairments their products are intended to cure or ameliorate, they also may have the effect of nor-malizing those impairments. Advertising is a way of making any particular condition open to discussion, of domesticating it and containing its effects: "Yes, you may have to urinate more frequently now, but don't be alarmed—lots of other people do too!" Viewers who may have been worried that they were the only one with their particular problem may come to feel more "normal" than before. Although the pressure exists for viewers to medicalize the workings of their bodies in ways designed to enrich the drug companies—advertising works, after all—those viewers could, alternatively, decide to support each other in resisting the false promise of eternal youth.

We could, for example, push to make changes in environments (for people of all ages) rather than in individuals (of all ages): We could make workplaces safer and schools more tolerant (Critser 254, 145). Along with environmental changes, we might change the way we evaluate problems and provide care, seeking collective solutions, not just individual ones. Moynihan and Cassels tell us that "in 2003 Americans spent 1.7 billion on just one osteoporosis drug to slow the loss of bone density—Fosamax—yet it's highly unlikely the nation spent a fraction of that on public awareness campaigns to try to prevent elderly people [from] falling" (141). We could take McRuer's stance of the "critically disabled" and fully acknowledge our always already incipient disability (95–97): Thus, when we are interpellated by drug ads as impaired, we might respond, "Yes, I am, but what of it?" In other words, we could finally acknowledge the humanity of disabled people, including ourselves.


CONCLUSION

Finally, I want to respond to a friend of mine who, in a conversation about this chapter, suggested that some of the pills advertised may actually help people. I do not wish to deny that. Lipitor and the other statins (used to reduce high cholesterol), for example, *do* apparently reduce the incidence of heart attacks in people with certain risk factors (Critser 192). Even the so-called lifestyle drugs undoubtedly have their adherents. Perhaps I am skeptical because I am just not arthritic enough (yet) to want to take

Celebrex (which, unlike Vioxx, is still on the market) or like sex with men well enough to care whether they take Viagra. And yet I must admit that there is a kind of ad that could seduce me completely. It would go like this: "Worried that your memory is failing? That your cognitive skills are in a state of decline? That soon you'll be as demented as your aging mom and dad? All is not lost! Take two doses of Mem-Save a day and you will stop memory loss in its tracks! Add one dose of Cog-Improve per day, and you may actually become smarter than before! (Side effects may include Weltschmerz, nausea, and the delusion that you have sold your soul to the devil.)"

I am sure that I would take my chances and risk the side effects—anything to keep those neurons firing, making new memories and allowing thoughts to flow. Here I catch myself in a possible inconsistency when I ask myself: Is the ability to make lesson plans to me as skating is to Dorothy Hamill? Are we unable to be ourselves without the capacity to perform the work that has come to define us? Possibly we all fear the loss of work-based identities in a culture that respects work and disrespects age.

Prescription drug advertising plays upon these fears and intensifies them—without always being able to alleviate them because the magic pill does not yet exist. Gains in the treatment of Alzheimer's, for example, have been modest. Current medications like Aricept ameliorate symptoms but do not stop the progression of the disease. Targeted at the middle-aged offspring of people with Alzheimer's, the current commercial for Aricept features a frail older man (who remains silent) while his daughter talks to us about caring for him. In this case, the ad seeks to associate the pill with the daughter's love, not with a cure. When the magic pill does come along, if it does—the one that will halt the disease in its tracks or, better still, prevent it altogether—will we really need aggressive advertising to understand its virtues? Meanwhile, as my sister, a nurse practitioner and psychotherapist, tells me and her clients, people with dementia are ordinary people, deserving of respect.

## NOTES

1. Greg Critser, *Generation Rx: How Drugs Are Altering American Lives, Minds, and Bodies* (Boston and New York: Houghton Mifflin, 2005), 52. Hereafter cited in text as Critser.

2. Ray Moynihan and Alan Cassels, *Selling Sickness: How the World's Biggest Pharmaceutical Companies Are Turning Us All into Patients* (New York: Nation Books, 2005), 42. Hereafter cited in text as Moynihan and Cassels.

3. Louis Althusser, "Ideology and Ideological State Apparatuses," in *Lenin and Philosophy and Other Essays*, trans. Ben Brewster (New York: Monthly Review Press, 1971), 174. Hereafter cited in text as Althusser.

4. Lennard J. Davis, *Bending over Backwards: Disability, Dismodernism, and Other Difficult Positions* (New York: New York UP, 2002), 50. Hereafter cited in text as Davis *BB*.

5. Robert McRuer, "Compulsory Able-Bodiedness and Queer/Disabled Existence," in Snyder, Brueggemann, and Garland-Thomson, *Disability Studies: Enabling the Humanities* (New York: MLA, 2002), 88-94. Hereafter cited in text as McRuer. McRuer cites Judith Butler, *Gender Trouble: Feminism and the Subversion of Identity*, (New York: Routledge, 1990), 122, and her "Imitation and Gender Insubordination," in *Insider/Out: Lesbian Theories, Gay Theories*, ed. Diana Fuss (New York: Routledge, 1991), 21, in developing his argument that able-bodiedness is a repeated performance that is "bound to fail" and in coining the phrase "ability trouble" to suggest "the inevitable impossibility, even as it is made compulsory, of an able-bodied identity" (93-94).

6. Lennard J. Davis, "Bodies of Difference: Politics, Disability, and Representation," in Snyder, Brueggemann, and Garland-Thomson, *Disabilities Studies*, 105. Hereafter cited in text as Davis *BD*.

7. Harlan Hahn, "Advertising the Acceptably Employable Image: Disability and Capitalism," in *The Disabilities Studies Reader*, ed. Lennard J. Davis (New York: Routledge, 1997), 178. Hereafter cited in text as Hahn.

8. Paul Darke, "Understanding Cinematic Representations of Disability," in *The Disability Reader: Social Science Perspective*, ed. Tom Shakespeare (London: Cassell, 1998), 181. Hereafter cited in text as Darke.

9. Rosemarie Garland-Thomson, *Extraordinary Bodies: Figuring Physical Disability in American Culture and Literature* (New York: Columbia University Press, 1997), 8. Hereafter cited in text as Garland-Thomson.

10. Michael Warner, "Normal and Normaller: Beyond Gay Marriage," 168-69 no. 87, *GLQ: A Journal of Lesbian and Gay Studies* 5, no. 2 (1999): 119-70.

11. Michael Warner, *The Trouble with Normal: Sex, Politics, and the Ethics of Queer Life* (Cambridge: Harvard UP, 1999), 60.

# Contributors

**Catherine Belling** is assistant professor of Medical Humanities and Bioethics at Northwestern University's Feinberg School of Medicine in Chicago. Her work has been published in *Literature and Medicine*, *Journal of Medical Humanities*, *Journal of Clinical Ethics*, and *Academic Medicine*, and in several edited collections.

**Jennifer L. Croissant** is associate professor in the Department of Women's Studies at the University of Arizona. Recent publications include co-authored works on female athletes and knee injuries, university-industry research relations, and forthcoming works for encyclopediae and handbooks on science, technology, and society.

**Catalina Florina Florescu** teaches in the Writing Program at Rutgers University. She has published numerous articles on the medical humanities, body criticism, and queer studies. Her work appears in *Fuzy Spaces* (Purdue University Press, 2002), *The Patient: Essays in the Medical Humanities* (Bucknell University Press, forthcoming), and *Proceedings of the Semiotic Society of America* (2007).

**Lisa Gabbert** is assistant professor of Folklore and American Studies at Utah State University. Her interests include modernity and social change, landscape and place, festival, and medical folklore. She has published articles in the *Journal of American Folklore*, *Western Folklore*, *Contemporary Legend*, and *Midwestern Folklore*, among others.

**Hayley Mitchell Haugen** is assistant professor of English at Ohio University, Southern, in Ironton, Ohio, where she teaches American literature and creative writing. Her work has appeared in *Cimarron*, *Columbia Magazine*, *The Charlotte Review*, *Kalliope*, *New Delta Review*, *Poetry Northwest*, *Rattle*, *Southern Poetry Review*, *Wordwrights*, and elsewhere, and she has written numerous nonfiction books for teens.

**Sally Hines** is a lecturer in sociology and social policy at the Centre for Interdisiplinary Gender Studies (CIGS) at the University of Leeds, UK. She is currently working on a project funded by the Economic and Socal Research Council (ESRC), which is examining recent legislative shifts around sexuality and gender. She has published articles in *The Journal of Gender Studies, Sociology, Critical Social Policy,* and *Sociological Research Online* as well as a number of chapters in edited volumes. Her book, *TransForming Gender: Transgender Practices of Identity, Intimacy and Care,* was published by Policy Press (2007).

**Stephen Johnson** is director of the Graduate Center for Study of Drama at the University of Toronto. His publications include *Roof Gardens of Broadway Theatres* and articles in a range of journals, including *The Drama Review, Canadian Theatre Review, Theatre Topics,* and *Nineteenth Century Theatre,* as well as *Theatre Research in Canada,* which he co-edited for ten years.

**Elizabeth Klaver** is professor of English at Southern Illinois University Carbondale. Her books include two monographs, *Sites of Autopsy in Contemporary Culture* (SUNY Press, 2005) and *Performing Television: Contemporary Drama and the Media Culture* (University of Wisconsin Press [The Popular Press], 2000). She edited the book *Images of the Corpse from the Renaissance to Cyberspace* (University of Wisconsin Press, 2004).

**Natalia Lizama** completed her PhD in the School of Social and Cultural Studies at the University of Western Australia. She is currently working on a project that examines the relationship between humans and animals in the context of anthropomorphism and zoomorphism. Her research interests include: the body, medicine, posthumanism, critical theory and postmodernism.

**Hillary M. Nunn** is associate professor of English at the University of Akron. She has published numerous articles on Renaissance drama. Her book *Staging Anatomies: Dissection and Tragedy in the Early Stuart Era* (Ashgate) appeared in 2005.

**Alexa A. Priddy** received her MA in Women's Studies from the University of Arizona in 2006. Her primary research interests are concerned with the medicalization of the body in contemporary discourses. She currently works for the Oregon Attorney General's Sexual Assault Task Force.

**Antonio Salud II**, M.D. and M.A., is a pulmonary and critical care medicine physician at Madison Medical Associates, Inc., in the Columbia-St. Mary's Community of Milwaukee, Wisconsin. He also serves as assistant clinical professor of medicine in the Department of Pulmonary Medicine and Critical Care and Population Health-Bioethics at the Medical College of Wisconsin. Dr. Salud is also trained in ethics.

**Linda Seidel** teaches English and women's studies at Truman State University. She is the author of "Leaving Caroline: The Social Construction of Motherhood in *A Proper Marriage*," *Re-Markings* 7, no. 1 (March 2008), a special issue on the work of Doris Lessing, and "Death and Transformation in J. M. Coetzee's *Disgrace*," *Journal of Colonialism and Colonial History* 2, no. 3 (Winter 2001).

**Sheena Sommers** is a doctoral candidate in the Department of History at the University of Toronto. She is a recipient of the Canada Graduate Scholarships Program Master's Scholarship and the Canadian Graduate Scholarships Program Doctoral Scholarship from the Social Sciences and Humanities Research Council of Canada. Her research interests include the history of the body, gender, and medicine in the eighteenth century.

# Index

able-bodiedness, 12; compulsory, 230-235, 236, 237; presentation, 238. *See also* McRuer, Robert

ableism, 230, 232, 233, 234, 236

absence, 113-114

*Absent Body, The*, 4, 10. *See also* Leder, Drew

advertising: celebrity endorsements in, 230; direct-to-consumer, 230, 231; of prescription drugs, 229, 230, 232, 233, 234, 236. *See also* Critser, Greg; Hamill, Dorothy

ageism, 230, 232, 236, 238, 240

agency, 1, 2; and constrained, 173, 177, 182, 188; and a woman's choice, 180, 181, 186-188. *See also* Lopez, Iris

Albala, Ken, 16, 17, 22, 31n10, 34n31, 34n42, 35n45, 35n49

Althusser, Louis, 231-232

Alzheimer's disease, 231, 240

anatomical museum, 2, 8, 9, 62-68; and abnormality, 63, 67, 77; and aesthetics, 63, 67, 81-82n4; audiences of, 63, 67; and authenticity, 62, 63, 66, 78; and bodily control, 62, 67-68, 73, 78, 80; characteristics of, 62-63, 65, 67, 81-82n4; and class, 67, 78; and gender, 63, 78; and instruction, 63, 65, 67, 82-

83n7; and medical profession, 65, 67-68, 83-84n11; and morality, 63, 67, 77; and race, 62, 65-66, 77, 78; relation to cabinet of 66-67; and sexuality, 65. *See also* Kahn, Reimers

anatomical Venus, 63, 82n5, 82n6

anatomy, 4, 5, 158, 162; abnormality, 127, 133; Act (England), 4; authenticity, 126, 133, 139-142; digital, 10; education, 128; normativity, 133; Renaissance, 3, 4

androgyny, 205

anesthesia, 163, 165, 167

Angelica, 21

animation, 129

anxiety, 152, 153, 155, 157, 163, 165

Apothecaries, Society of, 29

appetite, 15, 20-30

arthritis, 231, 233, 234, 239. *See also* Celebrex, Vioxx

arthroscopy, 162

Aston, Margaret, 30n1

Astra Zeneca, 238

*Atlas of the Visible Male*, 136, 143n19, 147n41. *See also* Spitzer, Victor and Whitlock, David

*At the Will of the Body*, 119. *See also* Frank, Arthur

authority, 153, 164

autonomy, 169

247